Treat Your Own Rotator Cuff

Jim Johnson, PT

Drawings by Eunice Johnson

First published by Dog Ear Publishing
4010 W. 86th Street, Ste H
Indianapolis, IN 46268
www.dogearpublishing.net

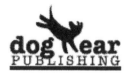

ISBN: 1-59858-206-2

This book is printed on acid-free paper.

Printed in the United States of America

How This Book Is Set Up

✓ Learn all about the rotator cuff in *Chapter 1*.

✓ Understand how rotator cuff exercises can fix shoulder problems in *Chapter 2*.

✓ Familiarize yourself with the rotator cuff exercises in *Chapter 3*.

✓ Pick the appropriate routine and begin in *Chapter 4*.

✓ Monitor your progress every few weeks with the tools in *Chapter 5*.

Contents

I have given my best effort to ensure that this book is entirely based upon scientific evidence and not on intuition, single case reports, opinions of authorities, anecdotal evidence, or unsystematic clinical observations. Where I do state my opinion in this book, it is directly stated as such.

—*Jim Johnson, P.T.*

1

What Exactly Is *a Rotator Cuff*?

Just imagine someone trying to follow a recipe for some brownies when they've never heard of flour. Be pretty hard, wouldn't it?

Well, the same thing would happen if I tried to explain the rotator cuff to you when you've never heard of a humerus or a greater tubercle–you'd be lost for sure! It is for this reason that we must first go over a little bit about the shape and structure of the shoulder, or what doctors refer to as your *shoulder anatomy*.

Don't worry though. If you're thinking that you'll have to commit to memory every last detail I'm going to cover in this section, you won't. Instead, all I really want you to do is just get a little familiar with the basic layout of the shoulder area and take in a few medical terms.

Armed with this knowledge, you will then be able to more clearly understand the rotator cuff, and more importantly, how to make it strong and keep it healthy.

The Shoulder Bones

Let's get started with a basic picture of the bones that make up the shoulder area (Figure 1.1):

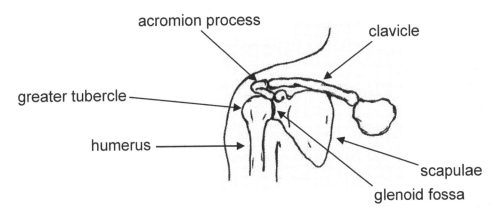

Figure 1.1 Looking at the right shoulder from the front–
the bones that make up the shoulder area.

As you can see, the shoulder is made up of many different bones, most with some pretty odd shapes. While they're all important in one way or another, we really need to be concerned with just *three* of them when learning about the rotator cuff.

The first one is known as the *humerus*, which is just a "funny" name for your upper arm bone. If you take another look at the above picture, you will notice a bumpy area at the end of it that bulges out. This particular part is known as the *greater tubercle*. You will find out shortly why this "big bump" is so important, but for now, just think of it as a hunk of bone that sticks out.

Next up we have the *scapulae*, or what most people call their shoulder blade. The scapulae is basically a triangular shaped bone with a couple of fingerlike projections poking out of one end. Pay particular attention to the one named the *acromion process* and the fact that is sits right over the humerus. Also notable is the *glenoid fossa*, which is a circular "crater" or socket that the humerus fits neatly into.

And last but not least, there's the *clavicle*, known to most of us as the collarbone. Oddly enough, it is the only bony connection between your arm and shoulder and the rest of your skeleton.

Although bones have many different functions, such as making blood cells and protecting vital organs, be aware that one of their main jobs is to provide firm places for the muscles to attach to.

The Shoulder Joints

Ever remember singing that song as a child, the one that goes "The foot bone's connected to the ankle bone..."? I'm betting most readers could still hum a few lines.

The point of this fun tune is that all the bones in our body are connected to each other and make up one big skeleton. In medical terms, the spot where two bones come together is known as a *joint*, and in the shoulder area, there are two important ones we need to talk about–the *gleno-humeral joint* and the *acromio-clavicular* joint. Here's an up-close look at them (Figure 1.2):

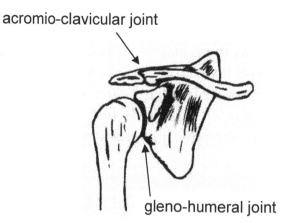

Figure 1.2 Looking at the right shoulder from the front
the gleno-humeral and acromio-clavicular (A/C) joint.

As you can see in the picture, the gleno-humeral joint is where the *glenoid* fossa of the scapula bone meets the *humerus* bone, hence the name gleno-humeral joint. And because the end of the humerus looks a lot like a ball, and the end of the scapulae looks a lot like a socket, many people refer to this type of joint as a *ball and socket* joint. True to their shape, ball and socket joints can quite easily rotate in many different directions, which in turn allows us to move our arms and legs all over the place.

While you do have other ball and socket joints in your body, the shoulder's gleno-humeral joint is just a little bit different. For comparison's sake, take a look at a picture of your right hip joint, which is also a ball and socket type joint (Figure 1.3):

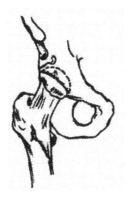

Figure 1.3 Looking at the right hip joint from
the front–a deep ball and socket joint.

Now glance back at *the shoulder's* ball and socket joint in Figure 1.2. See any differences? I'll bet you do, an obvious one being that the hip joint has a fairly deep socket, while the shoulder joint a pretty shallow one. Unfortunately, from a mechanical standpoint, this brings both good *and* bad news for our shoulders.

On the upside, the shoulder *is* able move around freely in many more directions than most of the other joints in your body such as the hip. This is simply because a shoulder "ball" can move quite easily in its *shallow* socket than the hip's "ball" can in its *deep* socket. But on the downside, all this great motion comes at a price, that being that it leaves the shoulder *very* vulnerable to slipping out of alignment–which is where a lot of shoulder problems begin.

As an example, researchers have found that even when the ball part of the joint slips only a few millimeters out of it's place, it's linked to shoulder problems (Deutsch, 1996). And, looking at the other end of the spectrum, it's not uncommon to hear of the ball coming *completely* out of its socket and dislocating, as in the case of a person falling to the ground with an outstretched arm. Either way, the fact of the matter is that when it comes to the shoulder's ball and socket joint, it's definitely a case of Mother Nature trading *stability* for *mobility.*

Now the last joint you'll need to be aware of is called the *acromio-clavicular joint* or *A/C joint* for short. In keeping with all the other joint names, the A/C joint gets its tongue-twisting title from the fact that it is formed by two bones, the *acromion process* of the scapulae (or shoulder blade) and the *clavicle* (or collarbone). Noteworthy because it sits right *above* the rotator cuff, the A/C joint too can dislocate, and when this happens, it is known as a *separated shoulder*.

The Rotator Cuff

Since you're now a little more familiar with the bones and joints of the shoulder area, we can begin to discuss the heart of the matter–the rotator cuff. Once again, let's start out with a simple picture:

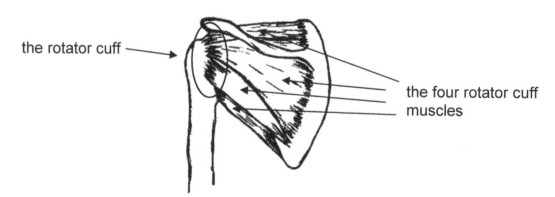

the rotator cuff

the four rotator cuff muscles

Figure 1.4 Looking at the left shoulder from behind–
the rotator cuff and the rotator cuff muscles.

As you can see, there are several arrows, one pointing to the rotator *cuff* and the others to the rotator cuff *muscles*. Although many people have a tendency to lump *all* of these structures together when they use the term "rotator cuff," know right off the bat that the rotator *cuff* is an entirely different kind of structure and tissue than the rotator cuff *muscles*.

The truth of the matter, and what a lot of people miss, is that the rotator cuff itself is really just a group of four flat **tendons** that fuse together and form a kind of "cuff" around the top part of your humerus. Since tendons connect the muscles to the bones, it's the job of the rotator cuff to help attach the rotator cuff muscles to the humerus. If any of this sounds a bit confusing, just remember that muscle connects to tendon, and tendon connects to bone– just like links in a chain. And the rotator cuff is *all* tendon.

The Rotator Cuff Muscles

If you counted them up in Figure 1.4, you found that there are no less than *four* rotator cuff muscles. Like the shoulder bones, scientists have also given the muscles some unusual names. They are:

- the supraspinatus
- the infraspinatus
- the teres minor
- the subscapularis

Clever readers will note that if you take the first letter of each muscle name and put them all together, they will actually spell out the word "SITS" –a little trick that has helped many a student remember them all on test day.

Now since most of the rotator cuff muscles are pretty different from one another and each have their own specific jobs, it's probably best if we take a brief look at them one by one.

Rotator Cuff Muscle Number One:
The Supraspinatus

Known for being the most frequently torn of all the rotator cuff muscles, the supraspinatus can be found on the *back* of your shoulder blade (Figure 1.5). It is here that it runs along the very top of this triangular bone and makes a straight shot to the greater tubercle, that "big bump" on your upper arm bone I pointed out earlier. Because it is buried under another muscle, as well as a bony part of the shoulder blade, it is hard to touch directly.

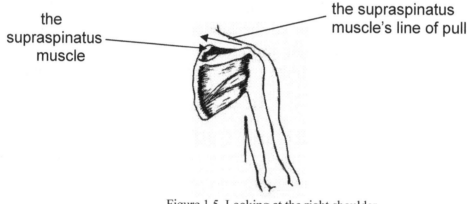

Figure 1.5 Looking at the right shoulder blade from the back–the supraspinatus muscle and its line of pull.

So what does the supraspinatus do anyway? Well, in order to figure out a muscles's function, researchers often look at what's called the "line of pull" of a muscle. Simply put, muscle fibers run in long, straight lines and pull on the bones when they contract By looking at the exact direction that they pull in, or their "line of pull," it can be determined which way a bone will move, the motion that will take place, and therefore what the muscle does. You can see the line of pull of the supraspinatus muscle represented by the top arrow in Figure 1.5.

Other clues can also be gotten by doing an *electromyographic* or *EMG study*. By inserting needles directly into the muscle of a subject and then asking them to move their shoulder around, the electrical activity of the muscle can be measured to see which motions the muscle is most active in.

Now as far as the job of the supraspinatus muscle, research has shown that its main task is to help you bring your arm out to the side, a motion referred to in medicine as *abduction* (Figure 1.6). Although the supraspinatus *is* very active in many other shoulder motions, abduction is considered its primary function.

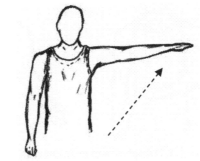

Figure 1.6 The supraspinatus muscle helps you raise your arm out to the side.

Rotator Cuff Muscles Two and Three: The Infraspinatus and Teres Minor

Figure 1.7 shows the next two rotator cuff muscles, the *infraspinatus* and *teres minor* muscles.

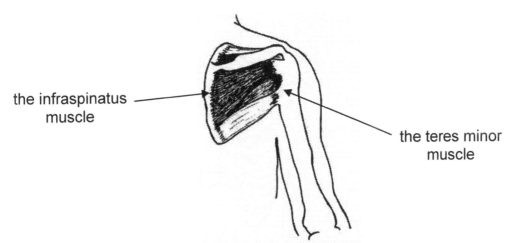

the infraspinatus muscle

the teres minor muscle

Figure 1.7 Looking at the right shoulder blade from the back–the infraspinatus and teres minor muscles.

As you can see, they sit right next to each other on the back of the shoulder blade. Because they both lie at the same angle and attach to the same area on the upper arm bone, they share the same job–to rotate your arm and shoulder *away* from your body. This motion is known as *external rotation*.

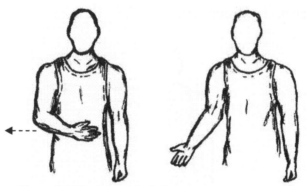

Figure 1.8 The job of the infraspinatus and teres minor muscles are to rotate your arm and shoulder *away* from your body.

Rotator Cuff Muscle Number Four: The Subscapularis

The biggest and strongest of all the rotator cuff muscles, the *subscapularis* can be found taking up the entire *front* of the shoulder blade (Figure 1.9).

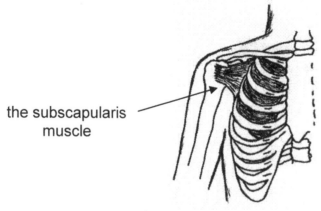

the subscapularis
muscle

Figure 1.9 Looking at the right chest area from the front. The subscapularis muscle is located on the *front* of the shoulder blade.

Like the teres minor and infraspinatus muscles, the subscapularis also helps you rotate your arm and shoulder around. However, instead of rotating them away from your body, the subscapularis is responsible for the exact opposite motion–rotating your arm and shoulder *towards* the body, a motion known as *internal rotation* (Figure 1.10).

The subscapularis gets this job because it attaches to the *front* of the upper arm bone, and not on the back, like the infraspinatus and teres minor muscles do. Here again, the spot where a muscle attaches to, as well as its line of pull, is very critical in determining what it will do.

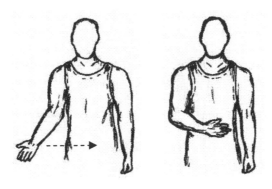

Figure 1.10 The job of the subscapularis is to rotate your arm and shoulder *towards* your body.

Why The Rotator Cuff Muscles Are So Important

Up to this point you've learned that the majority of the rotator cuff muscles help with *rotating* the shoulder–which is of course how they got their name. But while we've covered what each *individual* muscle does, I have yet to tell you about their most important job–what they do when they all work *together*.

Remember when we said that the shoulder is a ball and socket joint that is very mobile, yet very prone to coming out of place due to its shallow socket? Well, although nature has put our shoulders at a slight mechanical disadvantage, it didn't leave us totally helpless either. Instead of giving the shoulder a nice deep socket, like the hip joint, or lots of strong ligaments to hold the bones together, we've got the next best thing–powerful support from the rotator cuff muscles.

Individually, each of the four rotator cuff muscles have their own jobs. Some help roll the shoulder in, some help roll the shoulder out, and so on. But when all the rotator cuff muscles work *together* and contract at the same time, their combined pull helps keep the shoulder's ball and socket joint firmly in its place. Take a look at the line of pull of each individual rotator cuff muscle in Figure 1.11 and you'll see what I mean.

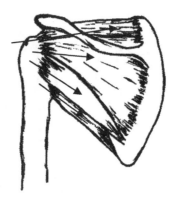

Figure 1.11 The lines of pull of the four rotator cuff muscles. When all of the rotator cuff muscles contract together, their combined forces hold the shoulder's ball and socket joint firmly in its place.

Each arrow in the above picture represents an angle that one of the four rotator cuff muscles is pulling in. As you can see, when the supraspinatus, infraspinatus, teres minor, and subscapularis muscles *all* contract at once, the net result is that the upper arm bone gets pulled snuggly towards the shoulder blade, thus firmly locking the "ball" into the "socket."

And when exactly does this happen, the rotator cuff muscles "kicking in" and contracting all at once to stabilize the shoulder joint? Well, according to the latest research, it occurs immediately *before* a person starts to move their shoulder around. For example, if you were to reach out right now and wave to someone, your rotator cuff muscles will contract the very instant *before* your arm actually starts to move. In this way, the shoulder joint starts out in a safe position and is held tightly in place as you go about using it. Pretty neat, huh?

Scientific-minded readers will also be glad to know that the research has confirmed the stabilizing role of the rotator cuff muscles. A study published in the peer-reviewed journal *Clinical Biomechanics* involved recording the EMG activity of people's shoulder muscles as they were asked to perform certain motions (David, 2000). Sure enough, researchers found that a "pre-setting" of the rotator cuff muscles occurred before any shoulder motion actually took place.

In a Nutshell

✓ The three important shoulder bones are the *humerus* (upper arm bone), the *scapulae* (shoulder blade), and the *clavicle* (your collarbone).

✓ The two important shoulder joints are the *acromio-clavicular joint* and the *gleno-humeral joint.*

✓ The gleno-humeral joint is a ball and socket type of joint and is prone to coming out of its place because of its shallow socket.

✓ The rotator cuff is a group of four flat tendons that fuse together and form a "cuff" around the top of your upper arm bone.

✓ The job of the rotator cuff is to connect the rotator cuff *muscles* to the top of your upper arm bone.

✓ The four rotator cuff muscles are the *supraspinatus*, the *infraspinatus*, the *teres minor*, and the *subscapularis.*

✓ The supraspinatus muscle helps you bring your arm out to the side.

✓ The infraspinatus and teres minor muscles help to roll your arm and shoulder *away* from your body.

✓ The subscapularis muscle helps to roll your arm and shoulder *towards* your body.

✓ The shoulder's ball and socket joint relies heavily on the rotator cuff muscles to stabilize it and keep it in its place.

✓ All the rotator cuff muscles contract at the same time *before* you start to move your shoulder in order to stabilize the joint as you use it.

2

The Many Shoulder Problems
This Book Can Help You Solve

While the exercises in this book can be used quite effectively to treat rotator cuff problems, their usefulness doesn't end there. Much research has accumulated over the years showing that when people get their rotator cuff muscles into shape, many other shoulder problems disappear as well. Therefore, the purpose of this chapter is to show you the many conditions that have been proven to get better when one "treats their own rotator cuff." But first, what exactly do I mean when I say *proven*?

The Randomized Controlled Trial

"Proven pain relief," say the television commercials. "Shown to be effective" reads the medicine bottle. It sounds good, and is exactly what people want to hear, but how do you *really* know it's true?

In a word, research. If you want to know if a treatment for a problem, any condition really, is truly effective, the *only* way you can know for sure is to find out the results of any studies that have tested out the treatment. And, if the study has been published in a peer-reviewed journal, meaning that other professionals in the field have read it first and think it is fit to print, all the better.

So what exactly should a person look for when digging around in the research? I mean in today's information age, there are literally *piles* of studies readily accessible to anybody.

Well, in medicine, we have what is known as *the randomized controlled trial*. This research method produces the highest form of proof showing whether or not a treatment really works and it's what you'll want to look for first, since it's the best of the best. Basically it goes something like this:

Say you want to prove that magnets get rid of shoulder pain. Well, first you would probably go out and find, maybe, 100 people that are having the same kind of shoulder pain and then *randomize* them into two groups of fifty–which means you pick them at random to be in one group or the other. Doing things this way keeps things fair because it makes sure that each subject has an equal chance at being put into either group–which makes sure that no one is purposely put here or there where they might do better or worse.

Next, you make one group the treatment group (meaning that they get to wear the magnets on their shoulders) and the other one a control group (meaning that they get no treatment at all). The control group is one of the most important parts of the randomized controlled trial as it lets you know how a person does all on their own, without any treatment, letting nature take its course.

Okay, so now you're ready to start your own randomized controlled trial and test out your theory that magnets do indeed get rid of shoulder pain. You give the people in the treatment group their magnets, let the people in the control group go about their normal business, and then check on everybody in, say, six weeks to see how their shoulder pain is doing. If, at the end of the six week trial, the magnet group has less pain than the control group, you can now say with confidence that magnets are indeed an effective treatment for shoulder pain. That's because everyone at the start of the study had the same kind of shoulder pain, an equal chance of getting into either group, and the group that wore the magnets were the only ones who got better. Therefore, we assume it must have been those magnets!

On the other hand, if the magnet group and control group both had the same amount of shoulder pain at the end of the six week study, then we would have to say that magnets *don't* work at all, simply because all subjects ended up with the same amount of shoulder pain whether they wore a magnet or not. Pretty nifty set-up, huh?

At this point, some readers might be wondering just why I'm dragging them through all this research mumbo-jumbo. Well, it's not because I'm trying to turn you into junior researchers or share my love of the scientific literature with you. No, it's for two *very* important reasons.

The first one is so that you can have every confidence that the stuff in this book really *does* work. Now that you know what a randomized controlled trial is, and that it produces the highest form of proof in medicine that a treatment is really effective, it will mean much more to you when I say that the exercises in this book have been shown in *numerous* randomized controlled trials to help out many different types of shoulder problems. Unfortunately, I doubt you'll find too many other books on the self-help bookshelf that can also make this claim.

The second reason I like to tell people about the randomized controlled trial is so that they will become more informed consumers. If you're like me, you work at least forty hours a week and quite possibly have a family to take care of. We all work hard for our money and I think it's really unfair when someone asks us to spend some of it on a product or service that makes miraculous claims without a shred of real evidence!

However, now that *you* know exactly what to look for when deciding on a treatment for a particular problem (one or more randomized controlled trials that show effectiveness), you'll be able to tell if it's something you want to invest your time and money in, or if it's clearly a hit or miss venture.

Conditions That Improve When You Treat The Rotator Cuff

The rest of this chapter is devoted to educating you in all the various shoulder problems that this book *can* help you with. While the exercises in the pages to follow cannot solve *every* shoulder problem, I think you'll find that they can tackle quite a few of the major ones. So, let's begin by taking a look at the number one shoulder problem that probably led most readers to pick up this book...

Shoulder Pain

Fresh out of physical therapy school, I thought I could fix the world. Armed with the latest medical knowledge, and a slew of neat little clinical tests, it seemed as though there would be no ache or pain I wouldn't be able to put a label on and fix. Unfortunately, later experiences proved otherwise.

While I found that I could pinpoint the cause of *many* patient's aches and pains, there would always be a few cases that left me scratching my head. At first I thought I was just a bad therapist or simply needed to read more literature. But then I realized one thing–medicine didn't have all the answers, so how could I?

I mean even though mankind did continue to make great gains in medical knowledge, testing, and technology each year, it had yet to figure out *all* the complexities of the human body. And until that day came, if it ever did, I'd just have to live with the fact that it would be unrealistic for me to think that I could put *every* patient's pain problem into a neat and tidy category.

Although disappointed, the whole issue did raise several interesting questions. While I might not be able to figure out the exact cause of some people's problems, should that necessarily keep me from getting them better? Sure it would be nice to know the precise source of everybody's pain, but do I necessarily *need* to know it in order to get them better?

I eventually decided "no" and reached this conclusion when I began using the treatment approach that pain is the end result of something not functioning properly, and so to make the pain go away, simply restore the function. As you can see, doing things this way solves several problems. It not only has the potential to get people better, but it does this *without* one having to know what the exact source of pain is.

To this day, and hundreds of patients later, I still use this approach. My initial evaluation is designed to gather information about the functioning of the problem area during which time I look at things such as what's strong, what's weak, or what's tight. Then, when I find something that's not working as it should, a treatment is given to the patient that is aimed at restoring the lost function. For example, if I find that your shoulder muscles are tight and you have trouble reaching around to touch the small of your back, you will get a stretching exercise to improve this motion.

Having said all that, you can now understand why I was quite delighted when I came across a randomized controlled trial that proved the usefulness of this approach. A study published in the peer-reviewed journal *Physical Therapy*, took sixty-six patients complaining of shoulder pain and aimed to get them better by improving the function of their rotator cuff muscles (Ginn 1997).

Patients in this study were excluded if their pain was in both shoulders, due to an inflammatory disorder or cancer, coming from the back, or because of an accident. Past that, it really didn't matter what the cause of the shoulder pain was in order for a patient to be included in the study, and in fact, some patients even had *no diagnosis*, meaning that the cause of their shoulder pain was unknown.

Now here's a few of the known diagnoses that patients *did* walk into the study with:

- tendinitis
- rotator cuff tear
- frozen shoulder
- osteoarthritis
- A/C joint problem
- biceps muscle tear

Typical of a randomized controlled trial, patients were put into either a treatment group or a control group. When reassessed one month later, follow-up results revealed that those who had restored the function of their rotator cuff muscles could move their shoulders with less pain, were more independent with daily personal care, and had a greater reduction in their shoulder symptoms. In stark contrast, the control group, which sat on a waiting list for a month without any treatment, got worse.

According to the results of this randomized controlled trial, improving shoulder function by treating the rotator cuff muscles is quite an effective way to fight shoulder pain, even in cases where the cause is *not* obvious.

Impingement Syndrome

At this point, most readers are probably thinking one of two things: "What the heck is impingement syndrome?" *or* "That's what I have!" In either case, I need to explain exactly what impingement syndrome is because I have known it to mean different things to different people. Sooo, let's start at square one.

When something is "impinged" it means that something is being squished between two things. If you've ever gotten your finger caught in a drawer or a doorway, your finger was being pinched or "impinged."

A similar thing can happen in the shoulder. This time, however, instead of your finger, it's your rotator cuff and a few other structures that can be pinched in an area known as the *subacromial space*. Here's where it's at:

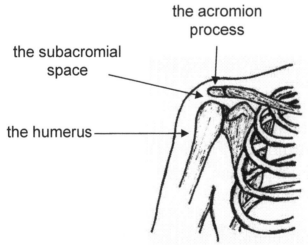

Figure 2.1 Looking at the right shoulder from the front–the subacromial space. In this space lies the rotator cuff as well as the subacromial bursa.

As you can see, the subacromial space is the area that lies *below* the acromion process, and *above* the humerus. Therefore, everything within this space sits right between two hard bones–which is precisely where the pinching or impingement can take place.

While many important structures can be pinched in the subacromial space, we're really concerned with just two in particular–the rotator cuff and something called *the subacromial bursa.* Since you're already a little familiar with the rotator cuff from the previous chapter, let's talk about the subacromial bursa for a moment.

Bursae in general are flat, sac-like structures that are located all throughout your body. If you've ever seen a deflated whoopie cushion, well, that's about what they look like. The shoulder's subacromial bursa is really no different than any of the other bursae, but since its home is right *below* the bony acromion process, it's called the *sub*acromial bursa.

Now it's the main job of these bursae to reduce friction and make things slide a whole lot easier, particularly in areas where structures have a tendency to rub together a lot–like when a tendon passes right over a bone. Normally they contain a small amount of fluid, however if they get irritated, they can really swell up and cause you a lot of pain. When this happens, doctor's call it *shoulder bursitis*, a condition I'm sure most readers have heard of before.

Having said all that, you now know what impingement is (something being pinched), where it takes place (the subacromial space), and what important structures get impinged (the rotator cuff and subacromial bursa). So, next we need to talk about *when* this problem can happen.

Figure 2.2 showns the subacromial space when your arm is hanging down at your side–a fairly good gap as you can see. Now take a look at Figure 2.3, which shows us what happens to the subacromial space *when you raise your arm up to use it.*

the subacromial
space

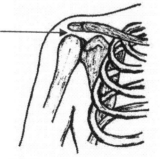

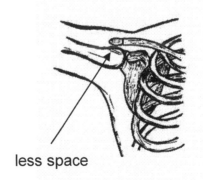

less space

Figure 2.2 The subacromial space when
your arm is hanging down at your side.

Figure 2.3 The subacromial space
when you raise your arm up to use it.

Wow! As you can see, the subacromial space does *not* always stay the same size. In fact, it gets *even smaller* when you raise your arm up. And just why is that? Well, largely because of the greater tubercle, that big bump on your upper arm bone I told you about earlier. Raising your arm brings the greater tubercle up and into the subacromial space where it takes up more room in an already crowded area–thus contributing to impingement of the rotator cuff tendons and bursa that sit directly above it.

At this point though, I need to make it perfectly clear that just because the subacromial space gets smaller when you raise your arm, that does *not* mean that the poor little rotator cuff and bursa are being brutally pinched all the time. As a matter of fact, in a normal state, when everything in the shoulder is functioning as it should, there is just enough room for all the structures in the subacromial space to carry on just fine *without* being impinged. However since space *is* limited and things are packed in there rather tightly, there's not much room for error either. So, when things do get out of whack and pinching does occur, you have what is called *impingement syndrome* (Figure 2.4).

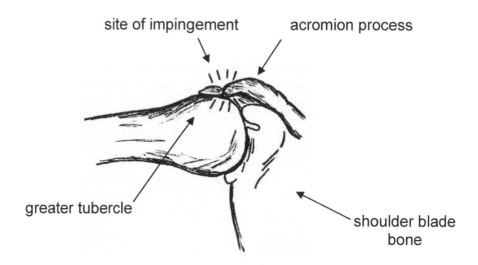

Figure 2.4 Looking at the right shoulder from the front. Impingement syndrome occurs when the subacromial bursa and rotator cuff get pinched between the acromion process and greater tubercle. This impingement happens as you raise up your arm.

The term "impingement syndrome" became popular in the early 70's when an orthopedic surgeon by the name of Charles Neer found a connection between torn rotator cuffs and acromion processes that had bony outgrowths or "hooks" on their tips (Figure 2.5).

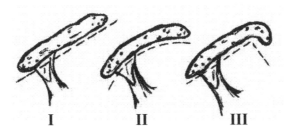

Figure 2.5 The three different types of acromion processes. Number three is known as a "hooked" acromion process and has been linked to impingement syndrome in several studies.

Based on these observations, Dr. Neer then proposed the theory that most rotator cuff tears were indeed caused by the tendons rubbing against the outer part of the acromion process, as well as the ligament that is attached to it (called the coraco-acromial ligament). Furthermore, he also found that the symptoms of impingement syndrome could be relieved in many cases by surgically cutting away part of the acromion process as well as its attached ligament. This procedure became known as the *anterior acromioplasty.*

Years later, another study came out that also showed a strong connection between "hooked" acromion processes and rotator cuff tears (Bigliani, 1986). The impingement theory eventually caught on and soon the anterior acromioplasty procedure became the treatment of choice for patients with impingement syndrome.

While it indeed seemed for a while that most rotator cuff tears were simply due to tendons mechanically rubbing on bone, later research began to crop up that raised some very serious questions as to the simplicity of Dr. Neer's original theory. For instance:

- studies also show that there are a lot of people with normal rotator cuffs, but *abnormal* acromion processes that *should* be causing wear and tear from impingement (Ozaki 1988, Ogata 1990).

- tears on the bottom part of the rotator cuff are much more common than tears facing the bony acrominon process (McConville 1999, Loehr 1987). If mechanical rubbing really was the cause of most tears, the side facing *towards* the bony acromion should show signs of wear first.

- randomized controlled trials show that patients with impingement syndrome can get better with just exercise (Brox, 1999). If the whole problem was just due to the tendons rubbing on bone, exercise wouldn't help patients with impingement syndrome since exercise doesn't change the shape of the bony acromion that is supposed to be the cause of the whole problem.

Today we know that rotator cuff tears are *not* all caused by a simple case of tendons rubbing on bone. Furthermore, the impingement syndrome can be divided into two distinct types:

- *primary impingement syndrome*–this is where the shoulder's "ball" stays firmly in its socket, but the rotator cuff and bursa are getting pinched because something is taking up extra room in the already crowded subacromial space (less room equals more of a chance that rubbing will occur). Some examples include bony spurring or an inflamed bursa.

- *secondary impingement syndrome*–this is where the rotator cuff and bursae are being pinched because there is a problem keeping the shoulder's "ball" centered in its socket. What happens here is that the "ball" slips *up* in the socket, thereby causing rubbing of the rotator cuff and bursae against the bony acromion process. Some reasons for this include having loose ligaments or rotator cuff muscle weakness.

Note that while each syndrome involves the rotator cuff and bursa rubbing against something and getting irritated, the reason *why* this occurs is entirely different for each syndrome. In primary impingement syndrome, the problem is that some structure is taking up extra room in the already narrow subacromial space. But, in secondary impingement syndrome, the problem is one of an unstable ball slippping up in its socket and causing the pinching. *The important point here is that while the end result of each syndrome looks the same–shoulder pain while raising your arm up due to pinching of the rotator cuff and bursa–the causes of each syndrome are entirely different.*

And that's precisely the reason why it's not good enough to just say that someone has shoulder pain due to "impingement syndrome." Instead, you really need to know *which* impingement syndrome a person has because the treatment for each is quite different. For example, someone with *primary* impingement syndrome may very well need surgery to remove a bony spur from their acromion process or A/C joint, while the person with *secondary* impingement syndrome may just need rotator cuff exercises to stabilize the "ball" part of the joint which is riding up and rubbing on the bony acromion process.

While diagnosing these two syndromes and learning how to tell them apart is beyond the scope of this book, let it be said that it requires a thorough work-up by a doctor which should include an MRI (magnetic resonance imaging) to get a good look at the soft tissues of the shoulder, as well as x-rays to view the the bones and subacromial space.

Now having given you the basics of impingement syndrome, the million dollar question still remains: can the exercises in this book effectively treat the two types?

Well, I've got some good news and some bad news for you on that one. The bad news is that if someone truly does have primary impingement syndrome, meaning that there is some structure crowding out the subacromial space, then the exercises in this book will probably *not* help you very much. This is because exercise *cannot*, for example, change or fix an arthritic spur.

However before you get *too* disappointed, let me also point out that most cases are probably *not* primary impingement syndromes. I say this because many randomized controlled trials have taken large groups of patients labelled with a general "impingement syndrome," treated them with rotator cuff exercises, and they got better compared to the control group. Therefore, most of the patients would have to have had a secondary impingement syndrome, simply because exercise can't fix a primary impingement problem for reasons discussed in the previous paragraph.

Three studies in particular support this notion. The first one (Brox, 1999), randomized 125 patients with "impingement syndrome" to one of three groups: a surgery group (removal of parts of the bursa, coracoacromial ligament and acromion process followed by shoulder exercises after surgery), an exercise group (exercises directed at the rotator cuff and shoulder), or a control group (a fake laser treatment).

Two and a half years later on long-term follow-up, the surgery group and the exercise group were doing much better than the control group, which of course tells us that surgery or exercise is better than doing nothing at all (no big surprise there). However what *is* pretty surprising is the fact that when these researchers looked at how the surgery group was doing compared to the exercise group, they discovered that each group was doing *the same* in terms of their pain, shoulder movements, strength, etc. Therefore, one can conclude from this randomized controlled trial with an exceptional follow-up period, that it makes no difference whether a patient has surgery to remove their acromion process or not for "impingement syndrome," as it seems to make little difference in how anybody does in the long run. The key, however, would appear to be the exercises involving the rotator cuff muscles which both treatment groups did get.

In a similar study (Haahr, 2005), ninety patients, once again with a non-specified type of impingement syndrome, were randomly assigned to either a surgery group (removal of parts of the bursa, coracoacromial ligament and acromion process followed by shoulder exercises after surgery), or an exercise group (scapular and rotator cuff muscle exercises). Follow-up one year later showed that both groups were doing the same, providing even more support to the idea that most impingement syndromes are of the secondary type. Remember that if most of the people in this study did have a *primary* impingement syndrome, the exercise group would not have done well at all since exercise alone cannot fix or change something like a bony spur rubbing on the rotator cuff in the prescence of a stable ball and socket joint.

And in a final study, researchers took a group of sixty-seven construction workers with "impingement syndrome" and randomly assigned them to either a control group, or an exercise group that strengthened their scapular and rotator cuff muscles (Ludewig, 2003). At risk of sounding like a broken record, the eight to twelve week follow-up period showed that those workers who exercised their rotator cuff muscles made significant improvements in pain and function, while the control group remained essentially the same.

While the results probably aren't shocking news to you by now, two things in this particular study are of interest. The first is the fact that the construction workers in the exercise group did their rotator cuff muscle exercises on their own, at home. They did *not* have anyone standing over them showing them exactly what to do every step of the way. This of course is good news to readers as it proves that it is entirely possible for one to get better and decrease shoulder pain with a simple set of exercises, not unlike the ones in this book. Other studies looking at the effectiveness of rotator cuff muscle exercises done at home have reached the same conclusion (Andersen, 1999).

Also, this particular study shows us what can happen to people with impingement syndrome when they let it go and don't treat it at all–it tends *not* to get better on its own. Just remember those construction workers in the control group that had no treatment at all–the condition of their shoulders remained the same over the study period.

So what's the real-world, bottom-line lesson here that these studies have to offer? Well, if you are unsure of which type of impingement syndrome you have (primary or secondary), give the exercises in this book a try. They've been shown in multiple, randomized controlled trials to help people who have been generally diagnosed with "impingement syndrome." And, if you get better, as most of the people in the studies have, it is quite likely that you suffered from a *secondary* impingement syndrome.

Tears of the Rotator Cuff Tendons

A fair amount of readers have probably been told that they have a "torn rotator cuff." If you do have one, or think you might have one, you probably have a million and one questions like most of the patients I've treated. Therefore, I'm going change things up a bit in this section and use a question and answer format to give you all the basics in a quick and concise manner. First up…

What is a rotator cuff?

We covered this in the first chapter, but it bears repeating just to make sure we're all on the same page. The rotator cuff is a group of four flat *tendons* that fuse together and form a kind of "cuff" around the top part of your upper arm bone. Since the job of a tendon is to connect muscle to bone, the rotator cuff links four rotator cuff *muscles* (the supraspinatus, infraspinatus, teres minor, and subscapularis) to your upper arm bone. These muscles help you rotate your shoulder around, lift your arm out to your side, and stabilize the shoulder's shallow ball and socket joint.

Sometimes when people use the term "rotator cuff," they are talking about the rotator cuff *and* the rotator cuff muscles as one, even though the rotator cuff is tendon and the rotator cuff muscles are muscle—two entirely different types of tissue.

What are the symptoms of a rotator cuff tear?

Symptoms of having a torn rotator cuff can vary widely from person to person and it is *never* a good idea to say for sure that somebody has a tear based upon any one, single symptom. Several studies have taken large groups of people with verified tears in their rotator cuff and evaluated how well their shoulders work (Duckworth 1999, Harryman 2003). Interestingly, both studies drew the same conclusion: the symptoms of a rotator cuff tear can vary *widely* from one person to the other. For example, some subjects said that they could lift eight pounds to their shoulder level or even throw a softball overhand twenty yards–while other subjects could not.

Keeping all this in mind, there are some symptoms that people with documented rotator cuff tears frequently (but not always) report:

- shoulder pain, commonly in the top, front, or side areas

- shoulder weakness which can limit activities such as combing your hair, tucking in your shirt, or putting dishes away. Reaching up above the level of the shoulder can be particularly troublesome.

- pain at night, especially when sleeping on the *same* side as the affected shoulder

How do doctors know if I've torn my rotator cuff?

Figuring out if you've torn your rotator cuff usually starts out with a history and physical or "H and P" in medical terminology. This would be where your doctor asks you questions and has a look at your shoulder. In many cases, this includes special tests that involve putting your shoulder in different postions to try and put stress on the rotator cuff. From all of this, it is impossible to be absolutely sure that you have a tear, although such an exam can lead to a strong suspicion.

Next, depending on your situation, additional imaging tests may be considered in order to get a "picture" of what's going on. Here are some common ones that doctors use:

- *an x-ray*, which looks mainly at the bony structure of your shoulder

- *an MRI*, which looks at the soft tissues (such as tendons and muscles)

- *an ultrasound*, which uses sound waves to create a picture of the inside of your shoulder

- *an arthrogram*, where a special dye is injected into your shoulder joint and then x-rays are taken. A normal rotator cuff should contain the dye within the joint, while a torn cuff allows dye to leak into the surrounding tissues.

After all is said and done, the information from the history and physical, as well as the results of any ordered imaging tests, are all put together to try and rule in or rule out a rotator cuff tear.

While this is a typical order of events that many people will go through in order to arrive at a diagnosis, this *may* vary depending on your particular doctor and situation.

Where exactly does the rotator cuff tear at?

Technically speaking, *any* of the four rotator cuff tendons could tear *anywhere*. However there are common patterns of tear, and the vast majority of them usually take place (or at least start out in) the very *top* part of the cuff that connects to the *supraspinatus* muscle (Tuite, 1998). Why is that you ask? Two reasons.

The first one has to do with the fact that the top part of the rotator cuff sits right between two hard bones. Being in such a position, it is at risk of being pinched and eventually frayed and torn as seen in the impingement syndrome we discussed earlier in the chapter.

The second reason has to do with the circulation that goes to the top part of the rotator cuff. Many research studies have conclusively shown that there is a very distinct area of the supraspinatus tendon (which is the top part of the rotator cuff) that doesn't have a very good blood supply at all (Determe 1996, Ling, 1990). This particular area of the rotator cuff has commonly become known as "the critical zone" (Figure 2.6).

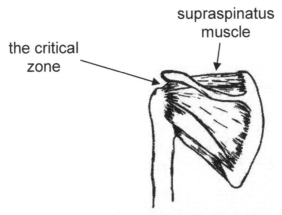

supraspinatus
muscle

the critical
zone

Figure 2.6 Looking at the left shoulder
from the back. Arrow points to the "critical
zone"–an area of the rotator cuff that has a poor
blood supply going to it. Also note that it
is located between two bones and is prone
to impingement as well. No wonder this is the
most frequently torn part of the rotator cuff.

Are there different kinds of rotator cuff tears?

Without question, all tears are not the same. Describing them, however, and putting them into neat little categories has proved to be a bit of a challenge. Many different classification systems have been proposed and in fact, about the only thing that can be agreed upon by researchers is that there is no perfect way yet to classify all the different kinds of tears. Having said that, there are some basic descriptions you'll commonly hear.

The first is known as a *full thickness tear* and is used when a rotator cuff tendon has been torn all the way through. You can compare this to poking a hole in a piece of paper with a pencil–the entire thickness of the paper has been torn completely through.

On the other hand, if the fibers of the rotator cuff tendon have been torn only part of the way through, it's referred to as a *partial thickness tear*. These kinds of tears commonly occur in one of three spots in the rotator cuff tendons and are named after the location of the tear (Figure 2.7).

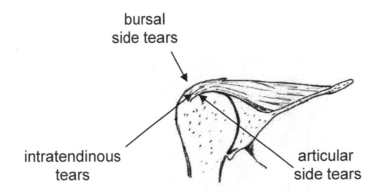

Figure 2.7 Looking at the right shoulder from the front. Arrows show the three locations where partial thickness rotator cuff tears commonly take place.

As you can see, bursal side tears occur on that part of the rotator cuff that faces the subacromial bursa (the top), articular side tears occur on that part of the rotator cuff that faces the joint (the bottom), and intratendinous tears occur *inside* the fibers of the rotator cuff (in the middle).

Can exercise help both partial and full thickness rotator cuff tears?

To my knowledge, the sad fact is that there have been no published randomized controlled trials yet to to prove *or* disprove the effectiveness of exercise to treat rotator cuff tears, full *or* partial thickness. Remember that the randomized controlled trial is the best of the best when it comes to proving whether or not a treatment for something is really effective and works.

However before you get too disappointed, also be aware that I have no trouble at all telling you that trying the exercises in this book will be *well* worth your while when it comes to treating *all* types of rotator cuff tears. This is because we have the next best thing to a randomized controlled trial for support–*multiple* consecutive case series studies showing that exercise *is* indeed effective for treating tears.

What is a consecutive case series study? Nothing fancy really. A good example would be an orthopedic surgeon taking his next 200 patients that walk through the door with a torn rotator cuff, treating them with exercises instead of surgery, and then re-evaluating them a year later to see how they all did. As you can see, it's not as good as a randomized controlled trial, one big disadvantage being the lack of a control group to compare things to. However since we do have *multiple* consecutive case series studies in the literature that consistently demonstrate the effectiveness of exercise to treat torn rotator cuffs, it is certainly reasonable to recommend it. And, *at the very least*, this level of support would certainly make exercise a very good option to try before considering something more invasive like surgery.

So what exactly do the published consecutive case series studies tell us? Well, for one, *home* exercise programs that emphasize stretching and strengthening the rotator cuff muscles can be *very* effective at treating tears (Wirth 1997, Goldberg 2001).

Other good news is that it appears that exercise will help you regardless of the size of your tear. For example, one consecutive case series study took a group of patients with documented rotator cuff tears and divided them up into partial defects, full thickness tears, or massive rotator cuff defects. All groups got the same home exercise program, and at the end of the twelve week study, *all* groups improved significantly (Heers, 2005).

What happens to a rotator cuff tear if I just leave it alone?

There's not a whole lot of research to tell us what happens to a rotator cuff tear that's left untreated. These kinds of studies are known as "natural history" studies and as of this writing, there is only one (Yamaguchi, 2001). In this study, researchers followed forty-five patients that had documented full thickness rotator cuff tears but *no* shoulder pain (yes, many studies have shown that you can have a torn rotator cuff and no pain, and nobody seems to know exactly how this can occur). Here's what they found:

- 51% of the subjects started getting shoulder pain during the follow-up period (which was between 3 to 8 years)

- 39% of the subjects that were recalled for repeat ultrasound examinations showed an *increase* in the size of the rotator cuff tear over time

- *none* of the patient's rotator cuff tears got smaller

From the available, limited evidence, it would appear that rotator cuff tears left untreated have a tendency to get worse over time. Hopefully more studies will follow that can tell us if different types of tears do better than others over the long run.

In a Nutshell

✓ **The randomized controlled trial is the highest form of proof in medicine that a treatment is effective and works.**

✓ **Rotator cuff exercises have been shown in randomized controlled trials to effectively treat shoulder pain and impingement syndrome.**

✓ **There are no randomized controlled trials yet to prove or disprove that exercise can effectively treat rotator cuff tears. There are, however, multiple consecutive case series studies showing that exercises help, which makes them a reasonable option to try.**

3

The Exercises

Now that you have been provided an overview of the rotator cuff and all the shoulder problems that can be solved by getting it into shape, it's time to move on to the heart of the book–the exercises that you can do in minutes a day to treat your own rotator cuff. Based entirely on the randomized controlled trials discussed in the last chapter, these exercises can be divided up into two very different types:

- *strengthening exercises*, which will make your muscles stronger

and

- *stretching exercises*, which will make your muscles more flexible

In this chapter, I'll be taking you step-by-step through each of the strengthening and stretching exercises so that you will know *exactly* how to do them. **Then, in the next chapter, we will put the exercises together into several routines to better suit your individual needs.**

The Stretching Exercises

While there are many different techniques to choose from when it comes to stretching out a tight muscle, by far the easiest and least complicated way is known as *the static stretch.* A static (or stationary) stretch takes a tight muscle, puts it in a lengthened position, and keeps it there for a certain period of time. For instance, if you wanted to use the static stretch technique to make the hamstring muscle on the back of your thigh more flexible, you could simply bend over with your knees straight and try to touch your toes. Thus, as you are holding this position, the muscle is being *statically stretched.* There's no bouncing, just a gentle, sustained stretch.

It sounds easy, perhaps a bit *too* easy, so you may be wondering at this point just how effective static stretching really is when it comes to making one more flexible. Well, a quick review of the stretching research pretty much lays it out straight as there are *multiple* randomized controlled trials clearly in agreement that we have a winning method on our hands. Here are the highlights:

- a study published in the journal *Physical Therapy* took 57 subjects and randomly divided them up into four groups (Bandy, 1994). The first group held their static stretch for a length of 15 seconds, the second group for 30 seconds, and the third for 60. The fourth group (the control group) did not stretch at all. All three groups performed *one* stretch a day, five days a week, for six weeks. Results showed that holding a stretch for a period of 30 seconds was just as effective at increasing flexibility as holding one for 60 seconds. Also, holding a stretch for a period of 30 seconds was much more effective than holding one for 15 seconds or (of course) not stretching at all.

- another randomized controlled trial done several years later (Bandy, 1997) set out to research not only the optimal length of time to hold a static stretch, but also the optimal number of times to do it. Ninety-three subjects were recruited and randomly placed into one of five groups: 1) perform three 1-minute stretches; 2) perform three 30-second stretches; 3) perform a 1-minute stretch; 4) perform a 30-second stretch; or 5) do no stretching at all (the control group). The results? Not so surprising was the fact that all groups that stretched became more flexible than the control group that didn't stretch. However what *was* surprising was the finding that among the groups that did stretch, no one group became more flexible than the other! In other words, the researchers found that as far as trying to become more flexible, it made no difference whether the stretching time was increased from 30 to 60 seconds, OR when the frequency was changed from doing one stretch a day to doing three stretches a day.

- additional randomized controlled trials have also supported the effectiveness of the 30-second stretch done one time a day, five days a week, to make one more flexible (Bandy, 1998).

As the randomized controlled trials clearly point out, it really doesn't take a lot of time to stretch out tight muscles *if* you know how. Based on the current published stretching research, this book recommends the following guidelines for the average person needing to stretch out a tight muscle with the static stretch technique:

- get into the starting position
- next, begin moving into the stretch position until a *gentle* stretch is felt
- once this position is achieved, hold for a full 30 seconds
- when the 30 seconds is up, *slowly* release the stretch
- do this one time a day, five days a week

One last note. While it is acceptable to feel a little discomfort while doing a stretch, it is *not* okay to be in pain. Do not force yourself to get into any stretching position, and by all means, skip the stretch entirely if it makes your pain worse.

Table Stretch

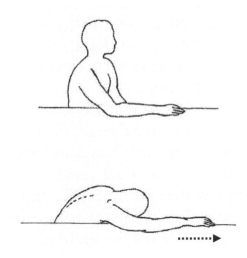

What's it for? Helps you to raise your arm over your head, a motion known as *flexion*.

How to do it: Sit down comfortably at a table in the same position as the the top picture. The arm you want to stretch should be the one on *top* of the table. Now, lean forward like the bottom picture, trying to "reach out" with your hand as far as you can until you feel a gentle stretch in the shoulder area. Hold for a full 30 seconds. The right shoulder is being stretched in the above picture.

Precautions: Do not force! This stretch in particular can *really* aggravate shoulders with an impingement problem or an irritated rotator cuff if you over do it. The goal here is to reach out and get a good stretch without experiencing ANY pain. If you can't get a gentle stretch in because it hurts too much, just work it forward as far as you can *without* pain.

Notes: This stretch works really well in the beginning stages of rehabilitating a shoulder because the stretch is performed on a table instead of you having to hold your arm up in the air against gravity. Just be patient. Over time, most patients are gradually able to reach out farther and farther, bit by bit.

Wall Walk

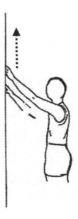

What's it for? Helps you to raise your arm over your head, a motion known as *flexion*.

How to do it: Stand facing a wall. Reach out and touch the wall at about the level of your waist to make sure you are starting out low. Next, "walk" your fingers straight up the wall until you feel a gentle stretch in the shoulder area. Hold for a full 30 seconds. The left shoulder is being stretched in the above picture.

Precautions: Do not force! This stretch in particular can *really* aggravate shoulders with an impingement problem or an irritated rotator cuff if you over do it. The goal here is to "walk" your fingers up the wall and get a good stretch without having ANY pain. If you can't get a gentle stretch in because it hurts too much, simply "walk" your fingers up the wall as far as you can *without* pain.

Notes: While this stretch does the same thing as the table stretch, it is a little more advanced because the shoulder is contracting its muscles in order to hold your arm up against gravity. Here again, be patient. Over time, most patients are gradually able to "walk" their fingers farther and farther up the wall, bit by bit.

Abduction Stretch

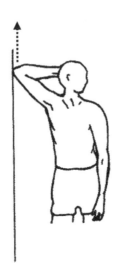

What's it for? Helps you to raise your arm over your head and out to the side, a motion known as *abduction*.

How to do it: Stand sideways against a wall just like the above picture. Now, slide your elbow straight up the wall until you feel a gentle stretch in the shoulder area. Hold for a full 30 seconds. The right shoulder is being stretched in the above picture.

Precautions: The main motion of the stretch is you sliding your elbow up the wall. Although it really doesn't matter what you do with your hand, make sure it is *behind* your head, not in front.

Notes: This stretch is a little more advanced since you already have to be able to raise your arm up above shoulder level to do it. It is a particularly good stretch for people who engage in activities or sports that require a lot of overhead motions.

Across the Chest Stretch

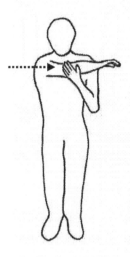

What's it for? Helps you to bring your arm across your body, a motion known as *horizontal adduction*.

How to do it: Stand up straight and put your hand on your elbow as in the above picture (the shoulder to be stretched goes across your body). Now, press your elbow to your chest/opposite shoulder until you feel a gentle stretch in the shoulder area. Hold for a full 30 seconds. The right shoulder is being stretched in the above picture.

Precautions: We want the arm being stretched (for example the right one in the above picture) to be at about shoulder level and no higher when you do the stretch. It is okay, however, to bring the arm *below* shoulder level a bit if raising it up that high hurts.

Notes: An especially good stretch to do if you have been told that you have tightness in your *posterior shoulder capsule*. The shoulder capsule is that tissue which surrounds the actual shoulder joint, and in some cases, it can become tight and limit a person being able to bring their arm across their chest.

Beginning Towel Stretch

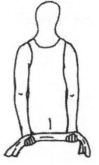 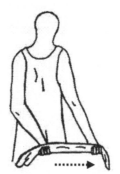

rear view of
starting position

rear view of
stretch position

What's it for? Helps you bring your arm behind your back, a motion
that makes your shoulder *internally* rotate. Therefore,
we're using this stretch to help improve *internal rotation* of
the shoulder.

How to do it: While standing up, grab a towel and hold it *behind* your back
like the picture on the left. Next, pull the towel out to the
side with the "good" arm (like the picture on the right) until
you feel a gentle stretch in the shoulder area. This sideways
motion will cause the hand of the tight shoulder (the left one
in the above picture) to be pulled towards the small of the
back, which in turn stretches out the shoulder. Hold for a full
30 seconds. The left shoulder is being stretched in the above
picture.

Precautions: Getting into this position can sometimes be tricky depending
on how irritated your rotator cuff is. Make sure you take the
time to *gently* ease your hand towards the small of your back.

Notes: Patients with a really irritated rotator cuff will hardly be able
to reach around at all when they first start this stretch.
However with every passing day or two, you will start to
notice that you can get your hand a little closer to the small of
your back. Once you are able to reach around and place your
hand over the small of your back, it is time to move on to the
Advanced Towel Stretch.

Advanced Towel Stretch

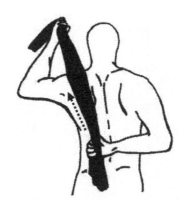

What's it for? Helps you bring your arm behind your back, a motion that makes your shoulder *internally* rotate. Therefore, we're using this stretch to help improve *internal rotation* of the shoulder.

How to do it: Grab a towel and get into the above position. With the "good" arm (the left one in the above picture), slowly pull the arm to be stretched up towards your head until you feel a gentle stretch in the shoulder area. Hold for a full 30 seconds. The right shoulder is being stretched in the above picture.

Precautions: Make sure you take the time to *slowly* and *gently* pull the hand up the back.

Notes: This is an advanced stretch that requires you to already be able to place your hand in the small of your back. If you can't do that, you will need to work with the **Beginning Towel Stretch** first until you can.

Doorway Twist Stretch

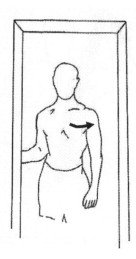

What's it for? Helps you to roll your arm out to the side, a motion known as *external rotation*.

How to do it: Stand in a doorway like the above picture, placing the arm you want to stretch against the wall/doorframe. Make sure that the hand, *as well as part of the wrist* is in contact with the wall. Next, rotate your body *away* from the arm that is touching the wall until you feel a gentle stretch in the shoulder area. Hold for a full 30 seconds. The right shoulder is being stretched in the above picture.

Precautions: In order to get a good stretch, make sure you keep your hand in its place and your elbow at a ninety-degree angle. This insures that the stretch takes place mainly at the shoulder.

Notes: A safe, beginning stretch that most shoulders should be able to tolerate.

Doorway Lean Stretch

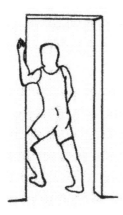

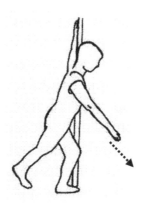

rear view of
starting position

side view of
stretch position

What's it for? Helps you to roll your arm out to the side, a motion known as *external rotation*.

How to do it: Stand in a doorway like the picture on the left. The arm you want to stretch is placed on the wall at shoulder level, with your elbow in an "L" position. Next, *slowly reach down in front of yourself* with the other arm, as if you are trying to pick something up off the floor a few feet in front of your body (like the picture on the right). Keep leaning directly towards the floor until you feel a gentle stretch in the front of your shoulder. Hold for a full 30 seconds. The left shoulder is being stretched in the above picture.

Precautions: Make sure that your forearm stays in contact with the wall throughout the stretch *and that you keep your elbow at a ninety-degree angle throughout the stretch.* This insures that the stretch takes place mainly at the shoulder. Also, it makes no difference which foot is in front of the other.

Notes: This is an advanced stretch that is especially useful to people who engage in activities or sports that require them to do a lot of overhead work. When done properly, it can dramatically increase external rotation.

The Strengthening Exercises

While the stretching exercises in the last few pages will make your shoulder muscles more *flexible*, it's the job of the strengthening exercises in this section to get them *stronger*.

But before jumping right in and going over all the exercises you'll ever need to beef up your rotator cuff, I think it's best to begin with a few strength-training basics. Because I wrote this book with *everyone's* rotator cuff in mind–from the bodybuilder who bench presses hundred of pounds, to the retired person who just wants to be able to pick up their grandkids–it's only wise to make be sure that we're all on the same page before going any further. Then, when we do get down to describing each of the strengthening exercises, every reader will know exactly what I mean when I say, "Do 1 set of 20."

So, using the handy question and answer format once again, let's start at the beginning….

How do we make a muscle stronger?

Muscles get stronger only when we constantly challenge them to do more than they're used to doing. Do the same amount and type of activity over and over again, and your muscles will *never* increase in strength. For example, if Karen goes to the gym and lifts a ten pound dumbbell up and down, ten times, workout after workout, week after week, her arms will *not* get any stronger by doing this exercise. Why? Because the human body is very efficient.

You see, right now, Karen's arm muscles can already do the job she is asking them to do (lift a ten pound dumbbell ten times). Therefore, why should they bother growing any stronger? I mean after all, stronger, bigger muscles *do* require more calories, nutrition and maintenance from the body. And since they can *already* do everything they're asked to do, increasing in size and demanding more from the rest of the body would only be a waste of resources for no good reason.

It makes perfect sense if you stop and think about it, but we can also use this same line of thinking when it comes to making our muscles bigger and stronger–we simply *give* them a reason to get into better shape. And how do we do that? By simply asking them to do *more* than they're used to doing. Going back to the above example, if Karen wants make her arm muscles stronger, then she could maybe switch from a ten pound dumbbell to a *twelve* pound dumbbell the next time she goes to work out. Whoa! Her arm muscles won't be ready for that at all–they were always used to working with that ten pound dumbbell. And so, they will have no choice but to get stronger now in order to meet the new demand Karen has placed on them.

For the more scientific minded readers, the physiology textbooks call this *progressive resistance exercise.* You can use this very same strategy to get *any* muscle in your body stronger, and we're certainly going to be using it to get your rotator cuff as strong as we can.

What's the difference between a repetition and a set?

As we've said, we need to constantly challenge our muscles in order to force them to get stronger and one good way to do this is to lift a heavier weight than we're used to using. Of course you won't always be able to lift a heavier and heavier weight *every* time you do an exercise, and so another option you have is to try to lift the same weight *more* times than you did before. As you can see, it's a good idea to keep track of things, just so you know for sure that you're actually making progress–and this is where the terms "set" and "repetition" come into play.

If you take a weight and lift it up and down over your head once, you could say that you have just done one repetition or "rep" of that exercise. Likewise, if you take the same weight and lift it up and down a total of ten times over your head, then you could say that you did ten repetitions of that exercise.

A set, on the other hand, is simply a bunch of repetitions done one after the other. Using our above example once again, if you lifted a weight ten times over your head, and then rested, you would have just done one set of ten repetitions. Pretty straightforward isn't it?

Now the last thing you need to know about reps and sets is how we go about writing them down. The most common method used, is to first write the number of sets you did of an exercise, followed by an "x", and then the number of repetitions you did. For example, if you were able to lift a weight over your head ten times and then rested, you would write down 1x10. This means that you did 1 set of 10 repetitions of that particular exercise. Likewise, if the next workout you did 12 repetitions, you would write 1x12.

*What's the best number of sets and repetitions to do
in order to make a muscle stronger?*

There was a time when I asked myself that same question. So, in order to find out, I completely searched the published strength training literature starting from the year 1960. I then sorted out just the randomized controlled trials, since they provide the highest form of proof in medicine that something is really effective, and laid them all out on my kitchen table. While getting to that point took me literally months and months of daily reading and hunting down articles, it was really the only way I could come up with an accurate, evidence-based answer.

Now the first conclusion I came to was that it is quite possible for a person to get significantly stronger by doing any one of a *wide* variety of set and repetition combinations. For instance, one study might show that one set of eight to twelve repetitions could make a person stronger compared to a non-exercising control group, but then again so could four sets of thirteen to fifteen reps in another study.

Realizing this, I decided to change my strategy a bit and set my sights on finding the most *efficient* number of sets and repetitions. In other words, how many sets and repetitions could produce the best strength gains with the least amount of effort? And so, I had two issues to resolve. The first one was, "Are multiple sets of an exercise better than doing just one set?" and the second, "Exactly how many repetitions will produce the best strength gains?"

Anxious to get to the bottom of things, I returned once again to my pile of randomized controlled trials, this time searching for more specific answers. Here's what I found as far as sets are concerned:

- the majority of randomized controlled trials show that *one* set of an exercise is just as good as doing *three* sets of an exercise (Starkey 1996, Reid 1987, Stowers 1983, Silvester 1982). This has been shown to be true in people who have just started weight training, as well in individuals who have been training for some time (Hass, 2000).

Wow. With a lot of my patients either having limited time to exercise or just hating it altogether, that was really good news. I could now tell them that based on strong evidence from many randomized controlled trials, all they needed to do was just *one set* of an exercise to get stronger–which would get them every bit as strong as doing three!

And the best number of repetitions to do? Well, that wasn't quite as cut and dried. The first thing I noted from the literature was that different numbers of repetitions have totally different training effects on the muscles. You see, it seems that the lower numbers of repetitions, say three or seven for example, train the muscles more for *strength*. On the other hand, the higher repetition numbers, such as twenty or twenty-five, tend to increase a muscle's *endurance* more than strength (endurance is where a muscle must repeatedly contract over and over for a long period of time such as when a person continuously moves their arms back and forth while vacuuming a rug for several minutes).

Another way to think about this is to simply imagine the repetition numbers sitting on a line. Repetitions that develop strength sit more toward the far left side of the line, and the number of repetitions that develop mainly endurance lie towards the right. Everything in the middle, therefore, would give you varying mixtures of both strength and endurance. The following is an example of this.

The Repetition Continuum

1 rep	10 reps	around 20 reps and higher

strength ——————————————→ endurance ——————→

Please note, however, that it's not like you won't gain *any* strength at all if you do an exercise for twenty repetitions or more. It's just that you'll gain mainly muscular endurance, and not near as much strength than if you would have done fewer repetitions (such as five or ten).

Okay, so now I knew there was a big difference between the lower repetitions and the higher repetitions. However one last question still stuck in my mind. Among the lower repetitions, are some better than others for gaining strength? For example, can I tell my patients that they will get stronger by doing one set of three or four repetitions as opposed to doing a set of nine or ten?

Well, it turns out that there really is no difference. For example, one randomized controlled trial had groups of exercisers do either three sets of 2-3 repetitions, three sets of 5-6 repetitions, or three sets of 9-10 repetitions (O'Shea, 1966). After six weeks of training, everyone improved in strength, *with no significant differences among the three groups.*

And so, with this last piece of information, my investigation had finally come to an end. After scrutinizing 45-plus years of strength training research, I could now make the following evidence-based conclusions:

- doing one set of an exercise is just as good as doing three sets of an exercise

- lower repetitions are best for building muscular strength, with no particular lower number being better than the others

- higher repetitions (around 20 or more) are best for building muscular endurance

In this book, we'll be taking full advantage of the above information by doing just one set of an exercise for ten to twenty repetitions. This means that you will use a weight that you can lift *at least* ten times in a row, and when you can lift it twenty times in good form, it's time to increase the weight a little to keep the progress going.

And why did I pick those numbers? Two reasons. The first has to do with the job of the rotator cuff. As you may recall, one of its main roles is to keep the shoulder's ball and socket joint firmly in its place. So, this means we need *stability*- but not only for quick tasks such as lifting a heavy box off the floor, but also for doing prolonged overhead work, such as changing a light bulb or painting a wall. Therefore, we're going to lean a little more towards the upper repetitions in order to boost the rotator cuff's endurance ability– while still staying low enough to substantially increase its strength. Remember, from around the twenty repetitions mark and up, you're going to gain mostly muscular endurance and a lot less strength.

The second reason? Well, it's a matter of safety. Using higher repetitions enables us to not only gain plenty of strength, but also use much *lighter* weights than if we'd chosen to work with the lower repetitions. This is because it takes a much heavier weight to tire a muscle out in, say, five repetitions, than it does to tire a muscle out in fifteen. And since most people would agree that you have a better chance of injuring yourself with a heavier weight as opposed to a lighter one, I recommend leaning more towards the upper repetitions.

How hard should I push it when I do a set?

How hard you push yourself while doing an exercise, also known as *exercise intensity*, is another issue that certainly deserves mention and is a question I am frequently asked by patients. The answer lies in two pieces of information:

1. Doing an exercise until no further repetitions can be done in good form is called *momentary muscular failure*. Research shows us that getting to momentary muscular failure or close to it produces the best strength gains.

2. You should not be in pain while exercising.

Taking the above information into consideration, I feel that a person should keep doing an exercise as long as it isn't painful and until no further repetitions can be done in good form within the repetition scheme.

Does it make any difference how fast you do a repetition?

Many randomized controlled trials have shown that as far as gaining strength is concerned, it does *not* matter whether you do a repetition fast or slow (Berger 1966, Palmieri 1987, Young 1993). Here's a look at one of the studies:

- subjects were randomly divided into three groups

- each group did one set of the bench press exercise, which was performed in 25 seconds

- the first group did 4 repetitions in 25 seconds, the second group did 8-10 repetitions in 25 seconds, and the third did 18-20 repetitions in 25 seconds

- at the end of eight weeks, *there were no significant differences in the amount of strength gained between any of the groups* (Berger, 1966)

So that's as far as strength is concerned. As far as safety, I recommend that you lift the weight up and down *smoothly* with each repetition, carefully avoiding any jerking motions.

A Quick Note on Isometric Exercise

The guidelines you've just read about apply to those type of strengthening exercises where your muscles contract while you're lifting a weight up and down. In exercise science, this type of exercise is known as *isotonic* exercise.

However what does one do if they need to strengthen their rotator cuff, *but they can barely move their arm at all?* Well if this is you, then rest easy. There is yet another proven way to strengthen your rotator cuff that involves very little arm motion. Impossible you say? Not really. It's called *isometric* exercise.

The word *isometric* comes from the two Greek words *isos*, meaning "equal" or "like," and *metron*, meaning measure. An isometric exercise, then, is one in which the length of the muscle stays the same as it is contracting. A good example of this is when you use your hand and arm to push hard against a brick wall. Your arm is still and unable to move because you can't push the wall over, yet, there is a definite building up of tension in your muscles that can be used as a type of resistance exercise.

But can something so simple as pushing on an immovable object *really* make one stronger? You bet it can. *Many* randomized controlled trials have proven beyond a shadow of a doubt that isometric exercise can greatly improve the strength of the big leg muscles (Maffiuletti 2001, Carolan 1992) as well as smaller upper body muscles (Grimby, 1973). In fact, some randomized controlled trials (Garfinkel, 1992) have even gone so far as to measure the cross sectional area of muscles with CT scans before and after isometric training–only to find that isometric exercise can actually make your muscles bigger!

With all this going for it, I've chosen to include a few isometric exercises in this book *specifically* for those readers who have such a painful shoulder that they can hardly lift it up or move it around at all. This would be, for example, someone who has recently torn their rotator cuff. The idea here is to start out with the isometric exercises and then eventually progress to the free weight exercises when your shoulder allows you to. By doing things this way, you will waste no time at all in getting your shoulder on the road to recovery.

So what exactly does isometric exercise involve anyway? Well, not much. The two in this book merely require a person to put their arm in a specific position, and then push their hand against a doorframe. Pretty easy, huh?

Now as far as how long and how many times you push, as well as how often, we'll once again be using evidence-based guidelines taken straight from multiple randomized controlled trials which have proven that isometrics can truly increase muscle size and strength. They are:

- push as hard as you comfortably can for 3 seconds
- repeat for a total of 30 times, once a day
- do this three times a week

And with this last bit of strength-training information, we're finished discussing the basics. So, now that we're all on the same page, let's move on to some of the best rotator cuff strengthening exercises medical research has to offer...

Isometric External Rotation

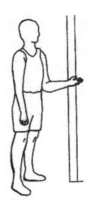

What's it for? Strengthens your rotator cuff muscles, particularly those that are involved in helping you rotate your arm and shoulder *away* from your body, a motion known as *external rotation*.

How to do it: Stand in a doorway and position yourself like the above picture. Make sure that the hand of the shoulder you want to strengthen is against the doorframe and that your elbow is bent at a ninety-degree angle. Now press against the doorframe as hard as you comfortably can with the back of your hand *for three full seconds.* Then, relax for a second or two and repeat. Do this for a total of thirty times in a row, once a day.

Precautions: It's okay to feel a little discomfort, but there should be no real pain to speak of as you're pressing against the doorframe.

Notes: It's okay to work up to the thirty repetitions if you can't do all thirty in a row the first time you try the exercise. For example, if you can only do twelve, shoot for doing thirteen or fourteen next time. Also, it doesn't really matter what you press against with the back of your hand, as long as your arm is in the same position as the picture. For instance, you could also do this exercise in sitting while pushing against an armrest.

Isometric Internal Rotation

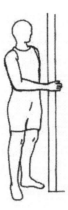

What's it for? Strengthens your rotator cuff muscles, particularly those
that are involved in helping you rotate your arm and shoulder
towards your body, a motion known as *internal rotation*.

How to do it: Stand in a doorway and position yourself like the above
picture. Make sure that the hand of the shoulder you want to
strengthen is against the doorframe and that your elbow is
bent at a ninety-degree angle. Now press into the doorframe
as hard as you comfortably can with the palm of your hand
for three full seconds. Then, relax for a second or two and
repeat. Do this for a total of thirty times in a row, once a day.

Precautions: It's okay to feel a little discomfort, but there should be no
real pain to speak of as you're pressing into the doorframe.

Notes: It's okay to work up to the thirty repetitions if you can't do all
thirty in a row the first time you try the exercise. For example,
if you can only do twelve, shoot for doing thirteen or fourteen
next time. Also, it doesn't really doesn't matter what you
press into with the palm of your hand, as long as your arm is
in the same position as the picture. For instance, you could
also do this exercise in sitting while pushing into an armrest.

Sidelying External Rotation

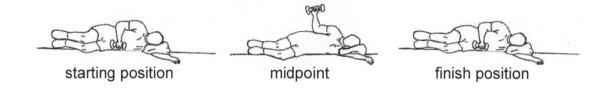

starting position   midpoint   finish position

What's it for? Strengthens your rotator cuff muscles, particularly those that are involved in helping you rotate your arm and shoulder *away* from your body, a motion known as *external rotation*.

How to do it: First, get in a comfortable position on your side, making sure that the shoulder you are going to strengthen is the one *on top*. Next, hold a dumbbell in your hand with your arm bent ninety-degrees at the elbow like the above pictures. Now smoothly lift the weight up as high as you comfortably can, making sure that you keep the ninety-degree bend in your elbow. Lower smoothly and repeat, working up to twenty times in a row, once a day.

Precautions: Make sure you're not rolling your body back as you do the exercise or lifting your *upper* arm off your body–it should stay on your side. Also, it's essential that you keep the ninety-degree bend in your elbow the entire time you're doing the exercise to make sure your rotator cuff is doing most of the work.

Notes: How high up you raise the weight towards the ceiling depends upon how irritated your rotator cuff is and how much tightness you have in your shoulder. Therefore, rather than worrying about raising your arm up to a set height, just concentrate on keeping your arm motion within a pain-free range. In time, chances are you'll notice that you will be able to lift your arm up higher and higher as you shoulder stretches out and becomes stronger.

Sidelying Internal Rotation

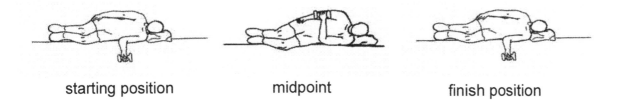

starting position   midpoint   finish position

What's it for? Strengthens your rotator cuff muscles, particularly those that are involved in helping you rotate your arm and shoulder *towards* your body, a motion known as *internal rotation.*

How to do it: First, get in a comfortable position on your side, making sure that the shoulder you are going to strengthen is the one *on the bottom.* Next, hold a dumbbell in your hand with your arm bent ninety-degrees at the elbow like the above pictures. Now smoothly lift the weight up as high as you comfortably can, making sure that you keep the ninety-degree bend in your elbow. Lower smoothly and repeat, working up to twenty times in a row, once a day.

Precautions: It's essential that you keep the ninety-degree bend in your elbow the entire time you're doing the exercise to make sure that your rotator cuff is doing most of the work.

Notes: Many studies have shown that exercise can effectively treat full thickness rotator cuff tears–and they usually include exercises to strengthen the *internal* rotators (Goldberg 2001, Wirth 1997, Hawkins 1995). Also, if you try this exercise and are uncomfortable lying on your hurt shoulder, you can use the **Alternative Internal Rotation–Standing** exercise on the next page instead.

Alternative Internal Rotation–Standing

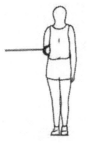 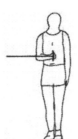 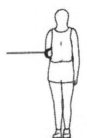

starting position   midpoint   finish position

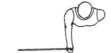 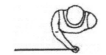 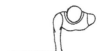

overhead view of   overhead view of   overhead view of
starting position   midpoint   finish position

What's it for? Strengthens your rotator cuff muscles, particularly those that are involved in helping you rotate your arm and shoulder *towards* your body, a motion known as *internal rotation.*

How to do it: Select the appropriate resistance (you can use a cable machine at the gym or elastic bands) and then get into the starting position as shown in the upper left picture. While keeping the elbow bent at a ninety-degree angle, *smoothly* pull the handle towards your body as far as you can comfortably go. Then, smoothly return to the starting position and repeat, working up to twenty times in a row, once a day.

Precautions: It's essential that you keep the ninety-degree bend in your elbow and your arm at your side the entire time you're doing the exercise to make sure that your rotator cuff is doing most of the work.

Notes: Use this exercise as an alternative if you've tried the **Sidelying Internal Rotation** exercise (previous page) and you're uncomfortable in that particular exercise position (lying on the affected shoulder).

Sidelying Abduction Exercise

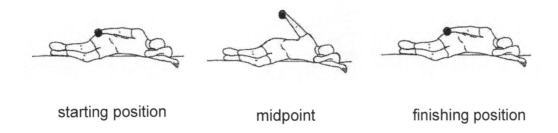

starting position   midpoint   finishing position

What's it for? Strengthens your rotator cuff muscles, particularly the *supraspinatus* muscle.

How to do it: First, get in a comfortable position on your side, making sure that the shoulder you are going to strengthen is the one *on the top*. Next, hold a dumbbell in your hand with your arm on your side like the far left picture. Now smoothly lift the weight up towards the ceiling, *going no higher than a forty-five degree angle* (as in the middle picture). Lower smoothly and repeat, working up to twenty times in a row, once a day.

Precautions: It's essential that you don't raise your arm up any higher than a forty-five degree angle when doing this exercise. Why? Going higher could cause impingement–which means pinching an irritated bursae or rotator cuff that is trying to heal.

Notes: This is one of the safest exercises you can do to strengthen your supraspinatus muscle–the most frequently torn of the four rotator cuff muscles.

Rowing Exercise

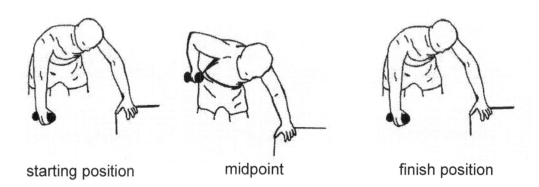

starting position   midpoint   finish position

What's it for? Strengthens the muscles that control and stabilize your
shoulder blade.

How to do it: First, find a sturdy object to lean on, such as a table-top.
Next, hold a dumbbell in the hand of the shoulder you want
to strengthen and get into the starting position (far left
picture). Now smoothly bend your elbow and pull the
dumbbell straight up to your side. Lower smoothly and
repeat, working up to twenty times in a row, once a day.

Precautions: Make sure that you bend over approximately forty-five
degrees like the above pictures. There's no need to bend over
more than that, but if you're not bent over far enough, the
shoulder blade muscles won't get worked adequately.

Notes: This one exercise works *many* of the muscles that control and
stabilize your scapulae (shoulder blade).

An Additional Note:

Why Work the Shoulder Blade Muscles if You Have a Problem with Your Rotator Cuff?

This is a good question patients often wonder about. Since the answer has a lot to do with how you move your arm, let's start out with a closer look at what exactly is happening as you reach up for something:

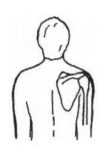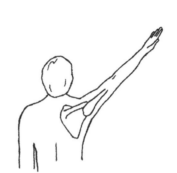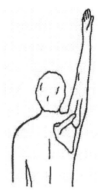

Figure 3.1 Looking at the right shoulder from the back. Note the resting position of the shoulder blade and upper arm bone.

Figure 3.2 As the arm is raised, note that not only has the upper arm bone moved, but so has the shoulder blade. Can you see that the shoulder blade has tilted up as the arm was raised?

Figure 3.3 Look at the shoulder blade now as the arm reaches way up. Compare this to the shoulder blade's original resting position in Fig. 3.1.

As you can see, reaching around and doing things involves a whole lot more than just your arm. Because your upper arm bone or *humerus* is attached directly to your shoulder blade, the two move in harmony as you use your arm to do things in various directions. In physical therapy school, I learned that this interaction is called your *scapulohumeral rhythm*. It's kind of a tongue twister, but just remember that all it really means is that as your upper arm bone is raised up, the shoulder blade comes along with it to varying degrees.

Now that you have that bit of knowledge, you can now see that the shoulder blade is really the "base of support" for the shoulder's ball and socket joint–which is exactly where the shoulder blade muscles come in– they are supposed to keep the shoulder blade *precisely* where it's suppose to be.

Here's a list of the major muscles that move the shoulder blade around as well as stabilize it:

- the rhomboids
- the trapezius muscle
- the levator scapulae
- the serratus anterior

All these muscles attach directly to your shoulder blade and when they are strong and doing what they're suppose to do, all is well–your shoulder joint has a stable base to work from, and the rotator cuff muscles can do their job without problems.

If, however, your shoulder blade muscles are weak or tire easily, the shoulder blade can start to move around abnormally and stir up trouble. For example, one MRI study (Solem-Bertoft, 1993) has shown that the more your shoulder blade starts to slip in a forward direction, the smaller the subacromial space gets–which in turn increases your chances of pinching the rotator cuff and bursae. Yet another interesting study (Ludewig, 2000) found that a group of subjects with symptoms of shoulder impingement had shoulder blades that failed to upwardly rotate properly when researchers asked them to raise their arms overhead.

So is the shoulder blade and how it moves important to the well being of our rotator cuffs? You betcha. Here's a diagram which summarizes the above ideas:

> ### *How Improperly Functioning Shoulder Blade Muscles Can Cause Shoulder Problems*
>
> **the shoulder blade muscles control
> and stabilize your shoulder blade**
>
> ↓
>
> **the shoulder blade is the base of
> support for your shoulder *joint***
>
> ↓
>
> **when shoulder blade muscles are weak
> or tire easily, they can cause the shoulder
> blade to move around abnormally**
>
> ↓
>
> **this can contribute to rotator cuff and
> other shoulder problems**

Exercise Validation

I've included this section just so you can have every confidence that the strengthening exercises I've selected for this book are indeed targeting and working *all* the right muscles. And, as always, I'll be citing you the published, peer-reviewed research to prove these claims.

Now there are two good ways researchers use to determine that an exercise does indeed work a particular muscle. The first is by using EMG or *electromyography*. This is where a needle or surface electrode is used to pick up the electrical signals that come from the muscle in order to tell just how active it is.

The second way is by MRI or *magnetic resonance imaging*. While most people think of MRI's as just being used to visualize the body's inner structures, such as the spinal cord or brain, few realize that it can also be quite useful to determine how active a muscle is, and in turn, which exercise works which muscle. Without getting too technical, exercise causes changes in the amount and distribution of water within a muscle, and since MRI's are able to detect these kinds of changes, they can be used as a good way to determine which muscle is working, and just how hard.

Below is a list of which strengthening exercises work which muscle(s), and the studies that have positively confirmed it. Please note that some of the studies have used MRI's, while others have used EMG's.

the exercise	*muscle that the exercise significantly activates*	*confirming studies*
isometric external rotation	**infraspinatus, teres minor**	**Reinold 2004**
isometric internal rotation	**upper and lower subscapularis**	**Suenaga 2003, Kadaba 1992**
sidelying external rotation	**infraspinatus, teres minor**	**Reinold 2004, Townsend 1991**
sidelying internal rotation	**upper and lower subscapularis**	**Decker 2003, Kronberg 1990**
alternative internal rotation–standing	**upper and lower subscapularis**	**Decker 2003**
sidelying abduction	**supraspinatus** **serratus anterior (mid and lower)**	**Horrigan 1999** **McMahon 1996, Moseley 1992**
rowing	**levator scapulae, rhomboids, trapezius (upper, mid, and lower)**	**Moseley 1992, Bradley 1991**

One last thing. When reading the list, be aware that any given exercise rarely works just *one* muscle. Therefore, the muscle you see listed under "*muscle that the exercise significantly activates*" is not the *only* rotator cuff muscle that is getting a workout when you do that particular exercise–others are kicking in as well. As an example, we're using the sidelying external rotation exercise to target the infraspinatus and teres minor muscles because EMG studies show that they are highly active when one does this particular exercise. Now the supraspinatus muscle is also active when doing this very same exercise, *but to a lesser degree*, and so we're using a different exercise, the sidelying abduction exercise, to target it a little better.

In a Nutshell

✓ **The exercises in this book consist of *stretching exercises* to make your muscles more flexible, and *strengthening exercises* to make them stronger.**

✓ **Multiple randomized controlled trials point out that muscles can be made more flexible by doing a static stretch for 30 seconds, one time an day, five days a week.**

✓ **Multiple randomized controlled trials point out that muscles can be adequately strengthened by doing one set of an exercise to momentary muscular failure.**

✓ **Lower repetitions have a tendency to increase a muscle's *strength,* while higher repetitions (around 20 or more) have more of a tendency to increase a muscle's *endurance.***

✓ **Multiple randomized controlled trials point out that isometric exercise is also capable of significantly increasing a muscle's size and strength by contracting the muscle as hard as comfortably possible for 3 seconds, thirty times a day, three days a week.**

4

Beginning, Intermediate, and Advanced Routines

The first exercise program I ever wrote for publication was in my book, *The Multifidus Back Pain Solution.* It consisted of three exercises, and I asked the reader to choose *only one.* The exercises were shown to be effective in randomized controlled trials, and if the diligent reader truly followed my specific, evidence-based guidelines, I could all but guarantee that their back pain would improve, if not go away altogether.

Eventually the book was translated into other languages, and as its popularity grew, I started getting some interesting feedback from worldwide readers. Two points consistently came up regarding the exercise routine:

- there weren't enough exercises in the book
- some of the exercises were too simple or they were ones that readers had already seen/done before

In case some of these same issues bother you as you review the exercise routines in this chapter, I would like to take a moment out to dispel a few common misconceptions. The first one is that some people think you have to spend a lot of time doing a lot of exercises in order to get better–which is simply untrue. If your exercise program is targeting the *correct* problem with *effective* exercises, then you should **not** be spending all day doing dozens of exercises. Of course there are exceptions, but they are few.

Another misconception is that simple, uncomplicated exercises are ineffective. Take stretching for example. Pulling your arm across your chest,
and holding it there for a mere thirty-seconds, once a day, may appear to some readers to be too simple a maneuver or too short a time frame to ever stretch out a tight muscle. But on the contrary, multiple randomized controlled trials have *consistently* pointed out that stretching for a longer period of time, or more times a day, will not produce better results.

And finally, the last common misconception deals with not trying an exercise because, "I've done that one before and it didn't help." The interesting thing I've noted is that when you question someone carefully about what they actually did, you often find that while a person may in fact have been doing an exercise correctly, they have *not* been following proper evidence-based guidelines. Using stretching as an example again, let's say that a person tries a particular stretch that is indeed targeting the correct tight muscle, only they've been holding the stretch for *fifteen-seconds* instead of the proven *thirty-seconds*.

After getting poor results for a period of time, most people will usually abandon the exercise and think, "That stretch didn't work." The truth, however, is that they really were doing a helpful exercise, it's just that they weren't following the correct evidence-based guidelines to make the exercise effective.

The moral? When proceeding with the exercises in this book, make sure that you do them *exactly* as instructed, even if you've tried some of them before or they seem too simple to be effective. Then and only then can you say with certainty that the exercises in this book were really helpful or not.

So, with that out of the way, I'm now going to answer some common questions that most patients usually ask when I go over an exercise routine with them–things like how much weight you should start off with or what equipment you'll need. After that, we'll move right into the three routines. Okay, first question…

How many times a week do I have to do the exercises?

There are two distinctly different kinds of exercises that make up the routines in this book–**stretching exercises** and **strengthening exercises**. In

Chapter Three, we covered the stretching literature and learned that in order to make a muscle longer, we need to stretch it for a full thirty-seconds, once a day, five days a week. Therefore, you will need to do the stretching exercises in each routine five out of seven days a week.

Now when it comes to the *strengthening* exercises, it's another matter entirely. Doing the same strengthening exercise every day, or even five days a week will usually lead to overtraining–which means *no* strength gains. Unlike the stretching exercises, muscles need more time to recover from the strengthening exercises, typically at least a day or so in between exercise bouts to rest and rebuild before you stress 'em again. And so, the question then becomes, which is better, one, two or three times a week?

Well, believe it or not, when I went through the strength training literature in search of the optimal number of times a week to do a strengthening exercise, there were a few randomized controlled trials actually showing that doing a strengthening exercise *once* a week was just as good as doing it two or three times a week. However, these studies were done on *very* specific populations (such as the elderly) or *very* specific muscle groups that were worked in a special manner (such as the low back muscles). Therefore, when you take this information, and couple it with the fact that there are a few randomized controlled trials showing that two and three times a week are far better than one time a week, there really isn't much support for the average person to do a strengthening exercise once a week to get stronger. And so, we're again left with another question of which is better, two versus three times a week–which is what much strength training research has investigated.

However it is at this point that the waters start to get a little muddy. If you take all the randomized controlled trials comparing two times a week to three times a week and lay them out on a table, you will get mixed results. In other words, there are some studies showing you that doing an exercise two times a week will get you the *same* results as three times a week, **but** there's also good research showing you that three times a week is *better* than two times a week. So what's one to do?

Well, in a case like this, the bottom line is that you can't really draw a firm conclusion one way or the other. So, you've got to work with what you've got. In this book, I'm going to recommend that you shoot for doing the strengthening exercises *three* times a week, because there is some good evidence that three times a week is better than two times a week (Braith, 1989). However, I'm also going to add that if you have an unbelievably busy week, or just plain forget to do the exercises, I'll settle for two times a week because there is also substantial evidence that working out two times a week is just as good as working out three times a week (Carroll 1998, DeMichele 1997).

So there you have it. While it may have been a whole lot easier to just answer the question by saying "do the stretching exercises five days a week and the strengthening exercises two to three times a week," I think it's good for readers to know *exactly* why they're doing the things I'm suggesting *and* that there's a good, evidence-based reason behind it.

What kind of equipment will I need to
treat my own rotator cuff?

Not much. The stretches require no equipment, so the only thing you'll need are some weights for the strengthening exercises. If you don't belong to a gym, the best option is to just go out and buy a set of dumbbells that are *adjustable*, meaning that you can change the plates on the end of them to turn them into a one pound dumbbell, or a two pound dumbbell, and so on.

Going out and buying a fixed one or two pound dumbbell, for example, is a mistake because once you can do an exercise for twenty repetitions with a one pound dumbbell, you will need to go out and buy a heavier dumbbell in order to keep getting stronger–which can get costly as you continue to move up on the weight. Adjustable dumbbells, on the other hand, are inexpensive *and* you can get them at just about any retail or sporting good store.

How much weight should I start off with?

For reasons we've already discussed in the exercise chapter, I recommend you shoot for doing one set of an exercise for ten to twenty repetitions. Therefore, you should start out with a weight that allows you to do a minimum of ten repetitions, but no more than twenty. But how do you figure that out?

Well, by trial and error. For example, let's say you begin trying the sidelying abduction exercise for the first time to strengthen your supraspinatus muscle. If you start out with a five pound dumbbell, but find you can do only six repetitions of the exercise, then the weight is too heavy–remember, we want you to choose a weight that you can do *at least* ten repetitions with. On the other hand, if you then try a one pound dumbbell, and are able to crank out thirty repetitions, the weight is way too light–this is because we want you to be able to use a weight that you can do *no more* than twenty repetitions with.

The next step, then, would be to try a weight between one and five pounds, say three pounds, and if you were able to do between ten and twenty reps with it, then that would be your starting weight.

While one, two, or three pounds may seem like a really light amount of weight for some readers to start off with, keep in mind that the rotator cuff muscles, unlike a lot of your arm and leg muscles, are pretty small and don't really require heavy weights in order to make them stronger. In fact, some people with a really bad tear in their rotator cuff might have to start out with *no* weight, just going through the motion of the exercises, while the majority of readers will probably start out with a weight that is less than ten pounds. Even very athletic or muscular patients that have fully rehabilitated their rotator cuff often find themselves using no more than around twenty pounds or so.

So always keep in mind that when it comes to strengthening your rotator cuff, the main idea is not to see how much weight you can lift, but rather to find a safe starting weight, and then *gradually progress* over time. Remember, when you can do twenty repetitions in good form, it's time to increase the weight by a pound or two to insure that the muscle keeps getting stronger.

Once I have strong rotator cuff, how do I keep it that way?

The research shows us that it takes only a fraction of the effort to *keep* the rotator cuff muscles strong than it took to get them that way. For instance, one randomized controlled took a group of subjects and had them do rotator cuff exercises three times a week for a total of twelve weeks (McCarrick, 2000).

With subject's rotator cuff muscles now a lot stronger at the end of the training period, investigators then set out to determine exactly how many times a week subjects would have to do their exercises in order to keep their newly gained strength. So, subjects were then randomly assigned to doing their rotator cuff exercises either twice a week, once a week, or not at all for *another* twelve-week period. At the end of this "reduced" training period, researchers re-checked everybody's rotator cuff strength and found that those subjects who trained at a frequency of one or two times a week showed *no* strength losses. Therefore, according to this study, if one has reached their goal and doesn't need to progress any further, all they need to do is exercise once a week to keep their strength gains–*as long as they are exercising at the same level of intensity each time.*

As a practical example of this, let's say that you worked up to twenty repetitions using a seven pound dumbbell with the sidelying abduction exercise. Your shoulder feels great, you can do what you need to do, and you have no need to strengthen it any further. So, since your "ending" weight and repetitions is using a seven pound dumbbell for twenty repetitions, you will need to continue lifting a seven pound dumbbell for twenty repetitions, once a week, in order to keep the intensity up and preserve your hard earned strength gains.

Note that you will *not* maintain your strength, for example, by doing *fifteen* repetitions with a seven pound dumbbell, or for that matter, doing twenty repetitions with a *five* pound dumbbell. Anything less than seven pounds for twenty repetitions is a *decrease* in intensity to your muscles–and if they don't have to do as much, they will certainly lose some strength.

*How do I fit rotator cuff exercises in
with the rest of my weight workout?*

If you regularly lift weights, I recommend that you consider modifying your workout in several ways:

- avoid doing any upper body exercises on the *injured* side that aggravate your shoulder. These are typically exercises that involve you raising your arm at or above shoulder level.

- if *every* upper body exercise you try to do on the injured side makes your shoulder hurt, skip working that side altogether.

- when you are basically symptom-free, it's okay to go ahead and test out those exercises again that previously aggravated your shoulder (such as those that involve you raising your arm at or above shoulder level). When you do, make sure you try them with *lighter* weights than you are normally accustomed to using. Over time, *gradually* increase the weight.

Above all, regardless if you are preventing a rotator cuff problem or rehabilitating one, it is important that you remember to do your rotator cuff exercises *last.*

The reason for this is that you don't want to be doing upper body exercises that stress the shoulder a lot with an *already* tired rotator cuff. This is exactly what will be happening if you fatigue the rotator cuff muscles first by directly exercising them *and then* do your upper body exercises.

How flexible do I need to get my shoulder?

A good question as I just hate it when people are given stretches to do but no clear guidelines as to when they need to stop. Let's first start out by looking at what is considered "normal" shoulder motion. Here's part of a list I found one time when I was looking into this matter:

source	shoulder flexion	shoulder external rotation	shoulder internal rotation
American Academy of Orthopaedic Surgeons (1965)	180°	90°	70°
Boone (1979)	167°	104°	69°
Esch (1974)	170°	90°	80°
Journal of the American Medical Association (1958)	150°	90°	40°
Kapandji (1970)	180°	80°	95°

As you can see by all the different numbers, there certainly seems to be a lot of confusion over what is considered "normal" shoulder motion. And why is that? Well, if you scrutinize the studies closely, the answer becomes obvious. Some studies measured *young* subjects, some *older* subjects, and some measured just *male* subjects. And to further complicate things, not all studies were even using the same method of measurement. No wonder it's so hard to sort things out! So, what do we do now?

Well, research was done once that measured four major shoulder motions in eighty-one normal subjects, aged 60 to 70 years of age, and calculated their average flexibility (Matsen, 1994). Therefore, given that you're not much over 70, I'm thinking that this would be a good *minimum* amount of shoulder motion for most readers to shoot for. After all, if a group of senior citizens have this much motion in their non-problematic aging shoulders, it's not unreasonable to expect that people younger than this should *at least* be this flexible.

Now the four major shoulder motions tested in this study were flexion, external rotation, internal rotation, and horizontal adduction. Since some of these motions I haven't explained and probably sound funny to most readers, here are some pictures showing each motion, how it's measured, as well as how much motion you should probably have as a minimum.

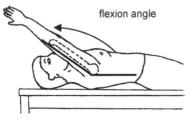

Motion: flexion
Minimum flexibility: 160° for males
167° for females

Note: A 0° angle would be lying on your back with your arm at your side, a 90° angle would be your arm pointing straight up to the ceiling, and a 180° angle would be when your arm is over your head and parallel to the floor. You can estimate your flexibility from these points. Get the help of an observer if you need to.

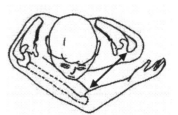

Motion: horizontal adduction
Minimum flexibility: 15 cm for males
14 cm for females

Note: Horizontal adduction is measured as the distance between your inner elbow and the bony bump on the front part of your shoulder (the acromion process). Use a tape measure and grab a buddy to get this measurement.

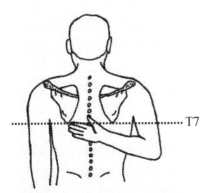

Motion: shoulder *internal* rotation
Minimum flexibility: T6 for males
                         T5 for females

Note: The T7 level is approximately
      the bottom tip of your shoulder
      blade. T6 is about 1/2 inch above
      T7. T5 is about one inch above T7.
      So, females should be able to touch
      about one inch higher than the bottom
      tip of the shoulder blade with their
      thumb, males, about half an inch.

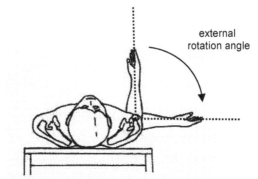

Motion: shoulder *external* rotation
Minimum flexibility: 72° for males
                         78° for females

Note: To check external rotation, lie on
      your back with your arm at your
      side. Now bend your elbow so that
      your fingers are pointing to the ceiling.
      Keeping your elbow in place, roll you
      hand out to your side. The above
      picture shows 90°of external rotation.
      Get the help of an observer if needed.

Once you've met the minimum flexibility standards for the four shoulder motions, it is up to you to decide if you need to keep stretching. If your shoulder is feeling fine and you have enough motion to do your day-to-day activities without difficulty, then you no longer have to stretch five days a week. At this point, doing the stretches one to two times a week should be enough to insure that you keep your current level of flexibility (please note that this number comes from my *clinical experience* rather than the research simply because there are too few studies done in this area to arrive at an evidence-based conclusion).

Now on the other hand, if you feel like you still have difficulty doing some activities because your shoulder is tight, or you just want more motion for certain athletic activities, simply continue stretching until you meet your goal. This would be cases, for example, where a worker does a lot of high, overhead activities and needs a bit more reach, or a baseball player who wants more external rotation for throwing the ball. Here again, after you've achieved your specific goal, I recommend stretching one to two times a week to keep your flexibility gains.

The Three Routines

Up to this point, we've built a good foundation of knowledge for you to be able to treat your own rotator cuff. With that accomplished, it's now time to pick a routine and get started. To do this, read through *all* three routines first, and then pick the one that best fits your particular situation. Then, refer back to Chapter 3 as needed for exercise instructions. And remember, don't forget to check with your doctor *before* starting any of the routines.

The Beginning Routine

Some people come to see me and they can hardly move their shoulder at all because it's so painful. If this sounds similar to your shoulder, then start with this routine. Move on to the Intermediate Routine and give those exercises a try when your shoulder motion improves and you can do the Beginning Routine without much discomfort. If you find that the exercises in the Intermediate Routine aggravate your shoulder, just go back to the Beginning Routine for a week and try switching again later. Repeat this process until you can tolerate doing the exercises in the Intermediate Routine.

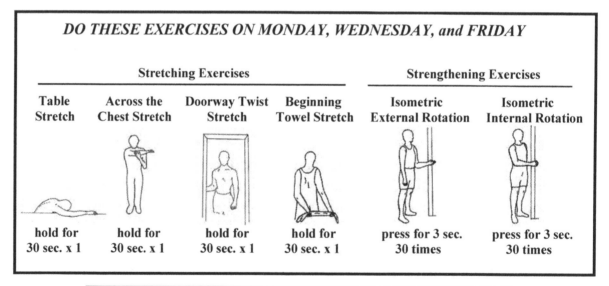

DO THESE EXERCISES ON MONDAY, WEDNESDAY, and FRIDAY

Stretching Exercises				Strengthening Exercises	
Table Stretch	Across the Chest Stretch	Doorway Twist Stretch	Beginning Towel Stretch	Isometric External Rotation	Isometric Internal Rotation
hold for 30 sec. x 1	hold for 30 sec. x 1	hold for 30 sec. x 1	hold for 30 sec. x 1	press for 3 sec. 30 times	press for 3 sec. 30 times

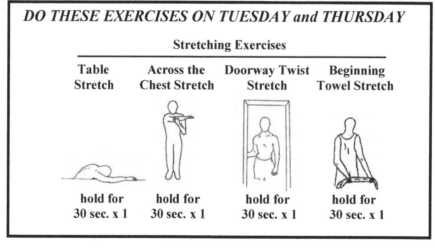

DO THESE EXERCISES ON TUESDAY and THURSDAY

Stretching Exercises			
Table Stretch	Across the Chest Stretch	Doorway Twist Stretch	Beginning Towel Stretch
hold for 30 sec. x 1	hold for 30 sec. x 1	hold for 30 sec. x 1	hold for 30 sec. x 1

The Intermediate Routine

Some people come to see me with a *moderate* amount of pain and *some* loss of shoulder motion. Although they can do a lot of normal activities, they do so with pain. If this sounds similar to your shoulder, begin with this routine (I suspect most readers will start with this one). Move on to the Advanced Routine and give those exercises a try when you can do the Intermediate Routine without much discomfort. If you find that the Advanced Routine aggravates your shoulder, just go back to the Intermediate Routine for a week and try switching again later. Repeat this process until you can tolerate doing the exercises in the Advanced Routine.

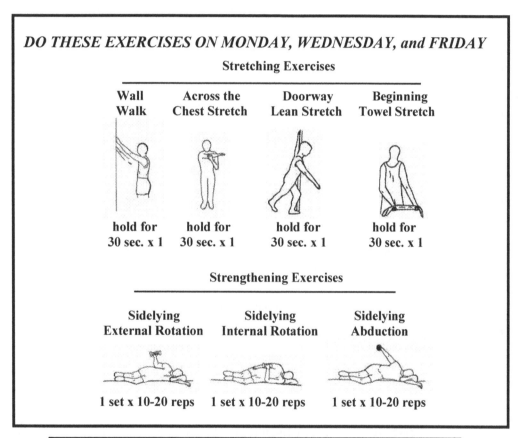

DO THESE EXERCISES ON MONDAY, WEDNESDAY, and FRIDAY

Stretching Exercises

Wall Walk	Across the Chest Stretch	Doorway Lean Stretch	Beginning Towel Stretch
hold for 30 sec. x 1	hold for 30 sec. x 1	hold for 30 sec. x 1	hold for 30 sec. x 1

Strengthening Exercises

Sidelying External Rotation	Sidelying Internal Rotation	Sidelying Abduction
1 set x 10-20 reps	1 set x 10-20 reps	1 set x 10-20 reps

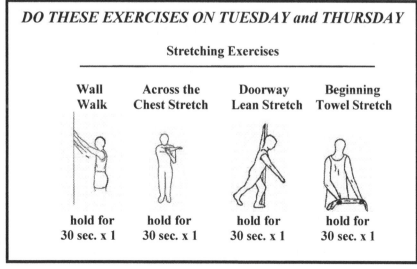

DO THESE EXERCISES ON TUESDAY and THURSDAY

Stretching Exercises

Wall Walk	Across the Chest Stretch	Doorway Lean Stretch	Beginning Towel Stretch
hold for 30 sec. x 1	hold for 30 sec. x 1	hold for 30 sec. x 1	hold for 30 sec. x 1

The Advanced Routine

Try this routine when you can do the exercises in the Intermediate Routine without much discomfort **or** if you are doing rotator cuff exercises to simply *prevent* a shoulder problem. While this routine includes a lot of the same exercises from the Intermediate Routine, it adds a very critical exercise for the scapular rotators, as well as several advanced stretches.

Over time, when you can do the Advanced Routine without difficulty, it then becomes your maintenance routine to preserve your hard earned gains. And remember, doing the stretches one or two times a week is usually enough to keep your *flexibility* gains, while doing one set of the strengthening exercises once a week is enough to preserve your *strength* gains.

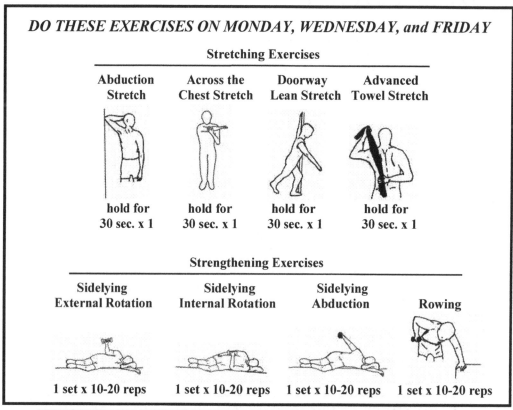

DO THESE EXERCISES ON MONDAY, WEDNESDAY, and FRIDAY

Stretching Exercises

Abduction Stretch	Across the Chest Stretch	Doorway Lean Stretch	Advanced Towel Stretch
hold for 30 sec. x 1	hold for 30 sec. x 1	hold for 30 sec. x 1	hold for 30 sec. x 1

Strengthening Exercises

Sidelying External Rotation	Sidelying Internal Rotation	Sidelying Abduction	Rowing
1 set x 10-20 reps	1 set x 10-20 reps	1 set x 10-20 reps	1 set x 10-20 reps

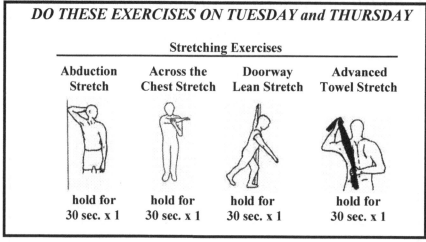

DO THESE EXERCISES ON TUESDAY and THURSDAY

Stretching Exercises

Abduction Stretch	Across the Chest Stretch	Doorway Lean Stretch	Advanced Towel Stretch
hold for 30 sec. x 1	hold for 30 sec. x 1	hold for 30 sec. x 1	hold for 30 sec. x 1

In a Nutshell

✓ A good therapeutic exercise program is one which targets the *correct* problem with *effective* exercises and should not keep you busy all day doing exercises.

✓ In many cases, simple, uncomplicated exercises work the best.

✓ Never say an exercise doesn't work until you've given it a decent try using good technique *and* evidence-based guidelines.

✓ Randomized controlled trials point out that stretching exercises should be done five times a week in order to make a muscle longer. Clinical experience indicates that stretching 1-2 times a week is enough to *preserve* flexibility gains.

✓ Randomized controlled trials point out that strengthening exercises should be done two to three times a week in order to make a muscle stronger, and that once a week is enough to *preserve* strength gains.

✓ A good way to strengthen safely and effectively is to start off with a weight that allows you to do at least 10 repetitions, but no more than 20.

✓ Do rotator cuff strengthening exercises *last* when fitting them in with the rest of your weight routine.

✓ How flexible you ultimately need to make your shoulder depends on what kind of activities you do. An athlete that does a lot of overhead motions, such as swinging a racquet, needs much more shoulder range of motion than a secretary with a sedentary lifestyle.

5

Measure Your Progress

Okay. You've learned all about the rotator cuff, picked a routine, started the exercises, and are on the road to recovery. So now what should you expect?

Well, we all know you should expect to get better. But what exactly does *better* mean? As a physical therapist treating patients, it means two distinct things to me:

- your shoulder starts to *feel* better

and

- your shoulder starts to *work* better

And so, when a patient returns for a follow-up visit, I will re-assess them, looking for specific changes in their shoulder **pain**, as well as their shoulder **function**.

In this book, I'm going to recommend that readers do the same thing periodically. Why? Simply because people in pain can't always see the progress they're making. For instance sometimes a person's shoulder pain is exactly the same, but they aren't aware that they can now actually do some motions or tasks that they couldn't do before–a sure sign that things are healing. *Or*, sometimes a person still has significant shoulder pain but they're not aware that it's actually occurring less frequently–yet another good indication that positive changes are taking place.

Whatever the case may be, if a person isn't looking at the big picture, and doesn't think they're getting any better, they're likely to get discouraged and stop doing their exercises altogether–even though they really might have been on the right track.

On the other hand though, what if you periodically check your progress and are keenly aware that your shoulder has made some changes for the better? What if you can *positively* see objective results? My guess is that you're going to be giving yourself a healthy dose of motivation to keep on truckin' with the exercises.

Having said that, I'm going to show you exactly what to check for from time to time so that you can monitor *all* the changes that are taking place in your shoulder. I call them "outcomes" and there are two of them.

Outcome #1:
Look for Changes in Your Pain

First of all, you should look for changes in your pain. I know this may sound silly, but sometimes it's my job to get a person to see that their pain *is* actually improving. You see, a lot of people come to physical therapy thinking they're going to be pain-free right away. Then, when they're not instantly better and still having pain, they often start to worry and become discouraged. Truth is, I have yet to put a patient on a rotator cuff routine and have them get instantly better. Better yes, but not *instantly* better.

Over the years, I have found that patients usually respond to rotator cuff exercises in a quite predictable pattern. One of three things will almost always occur as patients begin to turn the corner and become better:

- your shoulder pain will be just as intense as always, however now it is occurring much less frequently.

or

- your shoulder pain is now *less* intense, even though it is still occurring just as frequently.

or

- you start to notice less intense shoulder pain *and* it is now occurring less frequently

The point here is to make sure that you keep a sharp eye out for any of these three changes as you progress with the routines. If *any* of them occur, it will be a sure sign that the exercises are helping. You can then look forward to the pain gradually getting better, usually over the weeks to come.

Outcome #2:
Look for Changes in Shoulder Function

Looking at how well your shoulder works is very important because sometimes shoulder function improves *before* the pain does. For example, sometimes a patient will do the rotator cuff exercises for a while, and although their shoulder will still hurt a lot, they are able to do many things with their arm that they haven't been able to in a while–a really good indicator that healing is taking place *and* that the pain should be easing up soon.

While measuring your shoulder function may sound like a pain in the butt, it doesn't have to be. In this book, I'm recommending that readers use a quick and easy assessment tool known as *The Simple Shoulder Test* (Matsen, 1994).

The Simple Shoulder Test has actually been around for some time and is very well researched. Studies show that it is a valid test of shoulder function (Roddey 2000, Beaton 1996), has good test-retest reliability (Beaton, 1998), and is responsive to changes in shoulder function (Beaton, 1998). And best of all, it takes only a minute or two to complete. Now that's my kinda test!

So what exactly does taking the Simple Shoulder Test involve? Not much. You just read twelve questions, and check off either the "yes" or the "no" box, whichever answer applies best to your shoulder. Then, simply add up the number of "yes" boxes to see how many you have out of a possible twelve.

If you're wondering what a "normal" score is on the Simple Shoulder Test, it's when you have checked a "yes" to all twelve boxes (or a 12/12). We consider this "normal" because the researchers who developed the Simple Shoulder Test tested it out one time on eighty subjects between the ages of 60 and 70 whose shoulders were considered normal by history, physical examination, and expert shoulder ultrasound examination to exclude a rotator cuff tear. The results? *Essentially all subjects anwered "yes" to each of the test questions.* Therefore, providing you're not much over 70, a score of 12/12 is what you'll want to shoot for. On the next page is the test.

The Simple Shoot Test

	Yes	No

1. Is your shoulder comfortable with your arm at rest by your side? ☐ ☐

2. Does your shoulder allow you to sleep comfortably? ☐ ☐

3. Can you reach the small of your back to tuck in your shirt with your hand? ☐ ☐

4. Can you place your hand behind your head with the elbow straight out to the side? ☐ ☐

5. Can you place a coin on a shelf at the level of your shoulder without bending your elbow? ☐ ☐

6. Can you lift 1 pound (a full pint container) to the level of your shoulder without bending your elbow? ☐ ☐

7. Can you lift 8 pounds (a full gallon container) to the level of the top of your head without bending your elbow? ☐ ☐

8. Can you carry 20 pounds (a bag of potatoes) at your side with the affected extremity? ☐ ☐

9. Do you think you can toss a softball underhand 10 yards with the affected extremity? ☐ ☐

10. Do you think you can throw a softball overhand 20 yards with the affected extremity? ☐ ☐

11. Can you wash the back of your opposite shoulder with the affected extremity? ☐ ☐

12. Would your shoulder allow you to work full-time at your regular job? ☐ ☐

Now, write down how many "yes" boxes you checked out of 12 → ___ /12
The more out of 12 you have, the better, with 12/12 being a perfect score.

*The Simple Shoulder Test above is adapted from *Practical Evaluation and Management of the Shoulder (Matsen, 1994).*

So how did you do? Remember, the more "yes" answers you checked, the better. If you had twelve "yes" answers, you probably don't need this book too much. On the other hand, lower scores, such as 2/12 or 4/12, show much loss of shoulder function. If you did score this low, don't worry. Just keep taking the Simple Shoulder Test every few weeks, and as you progress with the exercises, you should see your score go up and up as time passes. Remember, sometimes shoulder function gets better *before* the pain does.

In a Nutshell

✓ **Being aware of your progress is an important part of treating your own rotator cuff–it motivates you to keep doing the exercises.**

✓ **Look for the pain to become less *intense*, less *frequent*, or both to let you know that the exercises are helping.**

✓ **Sometimes a shoulder starts to work better *before* it starts to feel better. Taking The Simple Shoulder Test from time to time makes you aware of improving shoulder function.**

References

Chapter 1

David G, et al. EMG and strength correlates of selected shoulder muscles during rotations of the glenohumeral joint. *Clinical Biomechanics* 2000;15:95-102.

Deutsch A, et. al. Radiologic measurement of superior displacement of the humeral humeral head in impingement syndrome. *J Shoulder Elbow Surgery* 1996;5:186-93.

Chapter 2

Anderson N, et. al. Self-training versus physiotherapist-supervised rehabilitation of the shoulder in patients treated with arthroscopic subacromial decompression: a clinical randomized study. *J Shoulder Elbow Surg* 1999;8:99-101.

Bigliani L, et al. The morphology of the acromion and its relationship to rotator cuff tears. *Orthopaedic Transactions* 1986;10:216.

Brox J, et al. Arthroscopic surgery versus supervised exercises in patients with rotator cuff disease (stage 2 impingement syndrome): a prospective, randomized, controlled study in 125 patients with a 2½ -year follow-up. *J Shoulder Elbow Surg* 1999;8:102-11.

Determe D, et. al. Anatomic study of the tendinous rotator cuff of the shoulder. *Surg Radiol Anat* 1996;18:195-200.

Duckworth D, et. al. Self-assessment questionnaires document substantial variability in the clinical expression of rotator cuff tears. *J Shoulder Elbow Surg* 1999;8:330-3.

Ginn K, et. al. A randomized, controlled clinical trial of a treatment for shoulder pain. *Physical Therapy* 1997;77:802-811.

Goldberg, B, et. al. Outcome of nonoperative management of full-thickness rotator cuff tears. *Clinical Orthopaedics and Related Research* 2001;382:99-107.

Haahr J.P., er al. Exercises versus arthroscopic decompression in patients with subacromial impingement: a randomized, controlled study in 90 cases with a one year follow up. *Ann Rheum Dis* 2005;64:760-764.

Harryman D, et. al. A prospective multipractice investigation of patients with full-thickness rotator cuff tears. The importance of comorbidities, practice, and other covariables on self-assessed shoulder function and health status. *Journal of Bone and Joint Surgery* 2003;85-A:690-696.

Heers G, et. al. Efficacy of home exercises for symptomatic rotator cuff tears in correlation to the size of the defect. Sportverl Sportschad 2005;19:22-27.

Ling, S.C., et. al. A study on the vascular supply of the supraspinatus tendon. *Surg Radiol Anat* 1990;12:161-165.

Loehr J.F., et al. The pathogenesis of degenerative rotator cuff tears. *Orthopaedic Transactions* 1987;11:237.

Ludewig P, et. al. Effects of a home exercise programme on shoulder pain and functional status in construction workers. *Occup Environ Med* 2003;60:841-849.

McConville, O, et. al. Partial-thickness tears of the rotator cuff: evaluation and management. *J Am Acad Orthop Surg* 1999;7:32-43.

Ogata S, et. al. Acromial enthesopathy and rotator cuff tear. A radiologic and histologic postmortem investigation of the coracoacromial arch. *Clinical Orthopaedics and Related Research* 1990;254:39-48.

Ozaki J, et al. Tears of the rotator cuff of the shoulder associated with pathological changes in the acromion. *Journal of Bone and Joint Surgery* 1988;70-A:1224-1230.

Tuite M, et. al. Anterior versus posterior, and rim-rent rotator cuff tears: prevalence and MR sensitivity. *Skeletal Radiol* 1998;27:237-243.

Wirth M, et al. Nonoperative management of full-thickness tears of the rotator cuff. *Orthopedic Clinics of North America* 1997;28:59-67.

Yamaguchi K, et. al. Natural history of asymptomatic rotator cuff tears: a longitudinal analysis of asymptomatic tears detected sonographically. *J Shoulder Elbow Surg* 2001;10:199-203.

Chapter 3

Bandy W, et. al. The effect of static stretch and dynamic range of motion training on the flexibility of the hamstring muscles. *Journal of Orthopaedic and Sports Physical Therapy* 1998;27:295-300.

Bandy W, et. al. The effect of time and frequency of static stretching on flexibility of the hamstring muscles. *Physical Therapy* 1997;77:1090-1096.

Bandy W, Irion J. The effect of time on static stretch on the flexibility of the hamstring muscles. *Physical Therapy* 1994;74:845-852.

Berger R, et. al. Effect of various repetitive rates in weight training on improvements in strength and endurance. *J Assoc Phys Mental Rehabil* 1966;20:205-207.

Bradley J, et. al. Electromyographic analysis of muscle action about the shoulder. *Clinics in Sports Medicine* 1991;10:789-805.

Carolan B, Cafarelli E. Adaptations in coactivation after isometric resistance training. *J Appl Physiol* 1992;73:911-917.

Decker M, et. al. Subscapularis muscle activity during selected rehabilitation exercises. *American Journal of Sports Medicine* 2003;31:126-134.

Garfinkel S, Cafarelli E. Relative changes in maximal force, EMG, and muscle cross-sectional area after isometric training. *Medicine and Science in Sports and Exercise* 1992;24:1220-1227.

Goldberg, B, et. al. Outcome of nonoperative management of full-thickness rotator cuff tears. *Clinical Orthopaedics and Related Research* 2001;382:99-107.

Grimby G, et. al. Muscle strength and endurance after training with repeated maximal isometric contraction. *Scan J Rehab Med* 1973;5:118-123.

Hass C, et. al. Single versus multiple sets in long-term recreational weightlifters. *Medicine and Science in Sports and Exercise* 2000;32:235-242.

Hawkins R, et. al. Nonoperative treatment of rotator cuff tears. *Clinical Orthopaedics and Related Research* 1995;321:178-188.

Horrigan J, et. al. Magnetic resonance imaging evaluation of muscle usage associated with three exercises for rotator cuff rehabilitation. *Medicine and Science in Sports and Exercise* 1999;31:1361-1366.

Kadaba M, et. al. Intramuscular wire electromyography of the subscapularis. *Journal of Orthopaedic Research* 1992;10:394-397.

Kronberg M, et. al. Muscle activity and coordination in the normal shoulder. An electromyographic study. *Clinical Orthopaedics and Related Research* 1990;257;76-85.

Ludewig P, Cook T. Alterations in shoulder kinematics and associated muscle activity in people with symptoms of shoulder impingement. *Physical Therapy* 2000;80:276-291.

Maffiuletti N, Martin A. Progressive versus rapid rate of contraction during 7 wk of isometric resistance training. *Medicine and Science in Sports and Exercise* 2001;33:1220-1227.

McMahon P, et. al. Comparative electromyographic analysis of shoulder muscles during planar motions: anterior glenohumeral instability versus normal. *J Shoulder Elbow Surg* 1996;5:118-23.

Moseley J, et. al. EMG analysis of the scapular muscles during a shoulder rehabilitation program. *American Journal of Sports Medicine* 1992;20:128-134.

O'Shea P. Effects of selected weight training programs on the development of strength and muscle hypertrophy. *Research Quarterly* 1966;37:95-102.

Palmieri G. Weight training and repetition speed. *Journal of Applied Sport Science Research* 1987;1:36-38.

Reid C, et. al. Weight training and strength, cardiorespiratory functioning and body composition of men. *Br J Sports Med* 1987;21:40-44.

Reinold M, et. al. Electromyographic analysis of the rotator cuff and deltoid musculature during common shoulder external rotation exercises. *Journal of Orthopaedic and Sports Physical Therapy* 2004;34:385-394.

Silvester L, et. al. The effect of variable resistance and free-weight training programs on strength and vertical jump. *Natl Strength Cond J* 1982;3:30-33.

Starkey D, et. al. Effect of resistance training volume on strength and muscle thickness. *Medicine and Science in Sports and Exercise* 1996;28:1311-1320.

Stowers T, et. al. The short-term effects of three different strength-power training methods. *Natl Strength Cond J* 1983;5:24-27.

Solem-Bertoft E, et. al. The influence of scapular retraction and protraction on the width of the subacromial space. An MRI study. *Clinical Orthopaedics and Related Research* 1993;296:99-103.

Suenaga N, et. al. Electromyographic analysis of internal rotational motion of the shoulder in various arm positions. *J Shoulder Elbow Surg* 2003;12:501-5.

Townsend H, et. al. Electromyographic analysis of the glenohumeral muscles during a baseball rehabilitation program. *American Journal of Sports Medicine* 1991;19:264-272.

Wirth M, et al. Nonoperative management of full-thickness tears of the rotator cuff. *Orthopedic Clinics of North America* 1997;28:59-67.

Young W, Bilby G. The effect of voluntary effort to influence speed of contraction on strength, muscular power, and hypertrophy development. *J of Strength and Conditioning Research* 1993;7:172-178.

Chapter 4

American Academy of Orthopaedic Surgeons 1965. *Joint motion: method of measuring and recording.* Chicago, AAOS.

Boone DC, et. al. Normal range of motion in male subjects. *J Bone Joint Surg* 1979;61A:756.

Braith R, et. al. Comparison of 2 vs 3 days/week of variable resistance training during 10- and 18- week programs. *Int J Sports Med* 1989;10:450-454.

Carroll T, et. al. Resistance training frequency: strength and myosin heavy chain responses to two and three bouts per week. *Eur J Appl Physiol* 1998;78:270-275.

DeMichele P, et. al. Isometric torso rotation strength: effect of training frequency on its development. *Arch Phys Med Rehabil* 1997;78:64-69.

Esch D, et. al. 1974. *Evaluation of joint motion: methods of measurement and recording.* Minneapolis: University of Minnesota Press.

Johnson, J 2002. *The Multifidus Back Pain Solution*. Oakland: New Harbinger Publications.

Journal of the American Medical Association 1958. *A guide to the evaluation of permanent impairment of the extremities and back*. JAMA (special edition) 1.

Kapandji I. 1970. *Physiology of the Joints Vols. 1 and 2, ed. 2*. London: Churchhill Livingstone.

Matsen F, et. al. 1994. *Practical evaluation and management of the shoulder*. Philadelphia: W.B. Saunders Company (p. 20).

McCarrick M.J., Kemp J.G. The effect of strength training and reduced training on rotator cuff musculature. *Clinical Biomechanics* 2000;15:S42-S45.

Chapter 5

Beaton D, et. al. Assessing the reliability and responsiveness of 5 shoulder questionnaires. *J Shoulder Elbow Surg* 1998;7:565-72.

Beaton D, et. al. Measuring function of the shoulder. A cross-sectional comparison of five questionnaires. *Journal of Bone and Joint Surgery* 1996;78-A;882-890.

Matsen F, et. al. 1994. *Practical evaluation and management of the shoulder*. Philadelphia: W.B. Saunders Company (p. 6).

Roddey T, et. al. Comparison of the University of California-Los Angeles Shoulder Scale and the Simple Shoulder Test with the Shoulder Pain and Disability Index: single-administration reliability and validity. *Physical Therapy* 2000;80:759-768.

Back Cover

Sher J, et. al. Abnormal findings on magnetic resonance images of asymptomatic shoulders. *Journal of Bone and Joint Surgery* 1995;77-A;10-15.

Yamanaka K, et. al. The joint side tear of the rotator cuff. A followup study by arthrography. *Clinical Orthopaedics and Related Research* 1994;304:68-73.

Lightning Source UK Ltd.
Milton Keynes UK
UKOW06f1837170215

246459UK00005B/344/P